THE CREATIVE SCREENWRITER

THE CREATIVE
SCREENWRITER

12 Rules to Follow— and Break—to Unlock Your Screenwriting Potential

Julian Hoxter

Illustration by Chris Gash

ROCKRIDGE
PRESS

Interior and Cover Designer: Michael Patti

Art Producer: Karen Williams

Editor: Erin Nelson

Production Editor: Matthew Burnett

Illustration © 2020 Chris Gash

ISBN: Print 978-1-64611-610-2 | eBook 978-1-64611-611-9

R0

To my students
in the School of
Cinema at
San Francisco
State University.

CONTENTS

Introduction

Screenwriting is an odd form of writing. It tries to communicate visually in ways that prose cannot. It speaks through movies and yet it hides itself behind them. The screenplay is the most important cog in the creative machine of film production, yet screenwriters often struggle to get the respect and remuneration they deserve. To be a screenwriter can be frustrating. Despite this, now is an exciting time to be a screenwriter. The media is changing, often in ways that are opening up possibilities for innovative writers to have their voices heard.

For my own part, I have been a screenwriter and a teacher of screenwriting for over 20 years. I have written independent features, produced documentaries, and written and edited academic studies of screenwriting as well as guides like this one. My own screenplays have won competitions and were finalists in many others. I frequently consult on independent screenplays, helping the writers develop their work toward production.

In my day job, I am on the faculty of the School of Cinema at San Francisco State University. I teach a diverse group of undergraduate and graduate cinema students who have a wide range of personal, professional, and creative goals. Happily, I love screenwriting, and I never cease to take great pleasure from helping my students and clients develop their scripts, whether they are mainstream genre movies or alternative, microbudget character dramas.

So, what about you? You might want to write the next Hollywood blockbuster or have secret ambitions to become an indie award show darling. Then again, maybe you want to write a very different kind of movie—one that looks and feels avant-garde. Whatever your aspiration, professional screenwriting is a hard and competitive business. That, of course, is what makes it exhilarating.

Beyond the talk of fame, recognition, and awards that span across genres, there is the creative process. Dedication to this creative process is the only thing you can truly rely on. And the process is what you have come to this book looking to hone.

You came here to learn more about screenwriting, so let's start by asking one of the most important questions: Who are you writing for? The immediate and most important answer should be *yourself*. If you are deeply invested in your own writing, you are more likely to have the dedication to shepherd a screenplay from first draft to completion—and through all the revisions that come with this enormous effort.

This book will help you understand what professional screenwriters do. The chapters here represent the "rules" or essential checkpoints you'll need to consider as you craft your work. While guidelines are listed plainly and simply, the point is also to assess them critically—to consider breaking or moving beyond them, when you have the confidence to do so.

How This Book Works

This book has a simple goal: to get you through your first (or next) screenplay. The book will walk you through the basic elements of screenwriting while giving you the permission and freedom to follow the rules when they suit you and abandon some of them when they don't. The elements here apply to all films—across every genre and for every budget—because the emphasis here is on *how* to write the thing, not *what* you finally produce.

If you are just starting out, I suggest you work through the steps of screenwriting in the order presented in the book. I wrote them in this order because this is what I have seen work best for a large number of students and respected screenwriters; the chapters build upon one another in a logical and systematic way. Indeed, the structure of the book is in itself a kind of lesson about process that you can learn just from following it. Of course, if you have more experience, feel free to dip in and out and use what is valuable in the way you see fit.

We will discuss the standard creative practices you need to know to get started, with plenty of examples to guide you along the way.

"Sage Spotlights" call out successful rule followers; "Breakout Stars" showcase the ideas of those who have forged their own path. Chapters also contain an "In the Writers' Room" exercise to deepen your understanding of the corresponding rule in the writing process. This is where you will put your ideas onto the page.

And so, as you build from one step to the next, you'll lay the bones of your work and better understand the creative challenge in front of you. Even if you don't sell your screenplay outright, the quality of your writing can get you noticed. Quality matters. And after you've finished reading the book, I hope you will return to it as a resource—for support when you wonder if you are doing the "right" thing, or for encouragement to redefine "right" altogether.

Before you launch into work on your screenplay, it's helpful to have a look at the industry that will shape your creative vision and your access to the screens that will hold your story.

SETTING THE STAGE

The good news is that, in some ways, the basics of movie stories haven't changed very much over the years: A character is still a character, a plot is still a plot. And yet as the industry changes, so do the stories that are sold and the way that they're told. This has to do with who has a seat at the table.

In Hollywood motion pictures, the producer and the studio executive wield the most creative control. Their priorities are making large profits, and they are looking for movies that can appeal to the widest audiences. Television, on the other hand, is much more of a writer's medium. In TV, the writers are often also the producers. This is especially true of TV made for digital platforms, where there is typically even more creative freedom than there is on legacy broadcast and cable networks.

Knowing what to expect from the industry can help you determine which levers to pull, who to talk to, and where you can find a home for your specific form of creativity. Let's allow the plot to unfold.

AN EVOLVING INDUSTRY

Today, there are more opportunities in the media for a diverse set of writers and other film artists than ever before. Still, when it comes to who has access, power dynamics are only beginning to shift. There is a long way to go to achieving equity in an industry long dominated by white, straight, cisgender men.

In the midst of this realignment, there has also been a seismic shift in the way people consume—and producers distribute—media content. The rise of streaming has transformed markets and content on both big screens and small. Streaming services like Netflix and Amazon Prime are producing an unprecedented amount of content—far more than the major Hollywood studios. The website Quartz calculated that in 2018, for example, Netflix alone produced around 1,500 hours of movies and series. Moreover, streaming services are now distributing movies in cinemas as well as online.

Importantly, major streaming platforms are allowing much greater flexibility to creatives. It is the writers and writer-producers who increasingly define what a series is, how long it should be, how an episode should work, or how unorthodox their one-off movies should be. In short, media outlets are *converging* and, right now, that is good news for screenwriters. Next, we'll take a look at the gatekeepers in the current media landscape. You can read this now to guide your script or return to this section once you have your finished product.

DIVERSITY BY THE NUMBERS

Inclusion in screenwriting can be looked at in a number of ways. One way is to look at the data. San Diego State University's Center for the Study of Women in Television and Film analyzes the top-grossing films each year; their report found that only 19 percent of the writers who worked on the 250 top movies of 2019 were female. Of those films, 73 percent had only male writers.

The Writers Guild of America West (WGAW) represents professional writers in motion pictures and television, and they also track diversity among their members. In the 2018–2019 season, the WGAW reported that in television, men took 61 percent of writing posts, while women held only 39 percent of those jobs. White writers held 73 percent of TV writer jobs, while only 27 percent went to writers of color. Higher-ranking TV writer jobs were held by an even more homogenous group: 76 percent of showrunners, who are in charge of writers' rooms, were men; 61 percent of showrunners were white. These statistics reflect decades of systemic inequality, and while they have improved (albeit at a glacial pace) over the past few decades, and especially these last few years, they are certainly not where they should be.

Hollywood Studios Are Thinking Globally

Many studios that were once independent are now owned by larger conglomerates. This means that making a million dollars on a good little movie is irrelevant when the corporation only values profits measured in hundreds of millions. As a consequence, the movies the studios green-light—or approve for production—need to have the potential to make a profit for other departments in the corporation. This can mean anything from physical media sales to branded products.

A studio's products are more likely to be co-productions, adaptations, or franchises. Studios are buying fewer original screenplays and are instead hiring writers for assignments. Additionally, major studios now care more about how their movies perform internationally because that's where the biggest box office sales come from.

This affects the way Hollywood movies are written. If a movie won't play abroad—i.e., if its style or content is too controversial for some markets, or if its story is complex and dialogue-driven—it is less likely to get the green light. Genres like fantasy and science fiction that used to be the province of B movies are now the A movies that drive studio profits. The genres that used to be A movies, especially dramas, are now largely the domain of independent cinema and streaming.

Yet it would be wrong to think that what defines movie production is genre. For one thing, not all big movies conform strictly to genre—just look at *Star Wars: Episode IV – A New Hope* (1977), which combined elements of the western, the samurai movie, and the weekly serial. And mainstream Hollywood doesn't own the old B movie genres, either.

No matter the scale of your story, as you're developing your screenplay, think about how it fits in the landscape of contemporary films, and how it might stand out.

Indie and "Indiewood"

As many of the old independent studios have gone under or been bought up by major studios, the boom in independent moviemaking has declined since its heyday in the 1980s and 1990s. Still, some of the big studios operate their own independent arms, like Disney's Searchlight Pictures (formerly Fox Searchlight). They tend to look for the kind of independent movie that they hope can cross over into the mainstream.

These days, movies made for studio subsidiaries, in which the distinctions between Hollywood and independent are blurred, are thought of as niche. Some critics refer to them as "Indiewood" rather than truly independent. For better or for worse, there is a kind of quirky formula to many of these Indiewood movies (think of *Garden State* [2004], among others).

THE INDIEWOOD FORMULA

What we really mean here is less a set of structural rules and more a set of stylistic approaches and attitudes to story. Most Indiewood movies tend to be more character-driven than mainstream genre pictures, but otherwise they follow the normal rules of Hollywood storytelling (perhaps with minor variation). Whereas Hollywood movies work hard to lose their audiences in the "reality" of their stories, watching an Indiewood movie can feel like we are sharing the poorly kept secret that we all know we are watching a movie and, what's more, we are feeling clever about knowing it. We can see this in stories as diverse as Wes Anderson's quirky family drama *The Royal Tenenbaums* (2001) and Olivia Wilde's buddy comedy *Booksmart* (2019).

Regardless of their production home, people are still making interesting and innovative films. There are also specialist genre producers out there, like Blumhouse, a company that focuses on horror movies. These producers allow writers to work in popular genres with smaller budgets. The market for smaller-budget movies has certainly changed, but a screenwriter with an innovative idea that's not a big action movie with franchise potential can still find the right producer, if they know where to look.

Streaming

Much of the best dramatic writing is now happening on TV. This is true for older networks and cable channels, as well as the newer streaming services like Netflix and Hulu.

Although this book is about feature screenwriting, much of its content also applies to episodic television writing. Some streaming series are breaking the rules of television and becoming more cinematized—looking toward movies, rather than old TV shows, for their style and rhythms of storytelling. This is something to bear in mind as you develop your story ideas, as they might have a home you weren't originally anticipating.

The question of whether a movie distributed by Netflix should "count" for Oscar consideration was raised for the first time by *Roma* (2018), and then by *The Irishman* (2019). As more talented people move from the big screen to expanded television, this trend is likely to grow, too.

Microbudget

Opportunities for writing and producing movies at very-low-to-no budget are better than ever. Avant-garde, political, risk-taking, and even simply broke filmmakers can get their movies made at this budgetary level, then get them seen more easily. Ava DuVernay started her film-making career with a short film, *Saturday Night Life* (2006), that had a budget of $6,000; later, she became the first black woman to direct a $100 million movie.

WHAT DO ALL MOVIES HAVE IN COMMON?

Let's bring this into focus: What is a story? At its most simple, a story is causality with a conclusion. In other words, it is a logical sequence of events that establishes a purpose and then resolves that purpose in some way.

There are different kinds of causal logic. Some are based on emotional connections rather than plot events, but even "non-causal" stories tend to follow some kind of logic. They are typically causal by another route. That's where things get complicated . . . and interesting. And it's precisely where you can get creative.

Why is causality so important? Without some kind of underlying system of connectivity, you don't really have a story because you don't have anything for us to *follow*. The pleasure we get from participating in storytelling, whether as a teller or as an audience member, is deeply connected with how our brains seek to make sense of the world. As a species, human beings are masters of pattern recognition, and we get deep pleasure from engaging in creative thinking. When you give us one piece of information, we are always seeking to know what else it might connect to.

The same goes for screenwriting. You show us that a character wants something, and we wonder how they might get what they want. We are already thinking ahead in your story, and already engaging with it. Whenever an event or some kind of change or development occurs in your story, we (your audience) are immediately trying to fit it into the context of what we already know and what we might be able to extrapolate in terms of possible outcomes.

In screenwriting terms, playing to the pleasure of pattern recognition is a vital part of *narration*. This is bound up in the process of storytelling, not just the story itself. Ever wondered why mysteries are a perennially popular genre? They have us follow clues and keep us guessing. In short, stories are deep human stuff.

Another way of thinking about this is through the idea of parallelism. Throughout the history of Hollywood, movies have told their stories through a kind of carnival mirror. What we establish in scenes and sequences in the first half of our movie becomes refracted and returned to us, changed but still recognizable, in the second half. In a Hollywood movie, characters change and develop, desires are fulfilled or left tragically unsatisfied, themes are enacted and resolved. In essence, the world of the story looks different at the end from how it looked at the beginning. If it doesn't—if the characters haven't changed and their actions have had no meaningful impact on their world—then, Hollywood usually asks, what was the point of your story?

In *Casablanca* (1942), the protagonist Rick Blaine—played by Humphrey Bogart—declares early in the movie: "I never stick my neck out for nobody." At the end of the film, not only has he stuck his neck out, but he has also re-committed himself to the world and to the struggle against fascism. He has been transformed by the events of the story and the pattern of his change is deeply resonant with the audience who has watched him earn his redemption.

Conversely, in another Humphrey Bogart picture, *In a Lonely Place* (1950), we are less engaged by character change as the marker of story resolution than we are by the causal logic of suspense. Dix, the screenwriter with anger issues played by Bogart, may have killed someone. His new love interest, Laurel, played by Gloria Grahame, grows terrified of Dix's propensity for violence, and she's disturbed by the unresolved question of the murder. In the end, another man admits to the killing, but Laurel leaves him. We understand why she leaves. Dix is cleared of the crime, but we leave him damaged and, as the movie title warns us, in a lonely place.

In other kinds of movies, change is measured in different ways. In the microbudget, character-driven movie *Hannah Takes the Stairs* (2007), a Joe Swanberg film, nothing much changes for the characters. Instead, the movie runs by its own emotional logic. A young woman named Hannah shuffles through a series of unsuccessful relationships and a bout of painful millennial self-critique, but at the end she bonds with a guy who is a fellow trumpet player. They serenade each other (rather poorly) in the bath, and that's a cute and possibly hopeful moment. What has really changed? Not a lot, and that's kind of the point.

In whatever way you conceive of, change, causality, patterns, and parallels are core storytelling elements. The job of every screenwriter is to create a story with a set of pictures that can evoke emotion. In this book, we focus on the core elements and key ideas that *every* screenwriter needs to understand in order to develop their writing. As the movie mogul Jack Lipnick says to the screenwriter protagonist in the Coen brothers' dark Hollywood comedy, *Barton Fink* (1991): "We're only interested in one thing, Bart. Can you tell a story? Can you make us laugh? Can you make us cry? Can you make us want to break out in joyous song? Is that more than one thing? Okay!"

HOLLYWOOD JARGON

What follows is a list of terms that you will need to be aware of in your screenwriting career. Many of them will come up again (and again) in the rest of the book, but even those that don't will be useful to you as you research, plan, write, and encounter people who work in movie development and production.

AGENT

Agents make deals. If you have a deal to make, you'll probably find an agent. If you have no connections and no real track record—in other words, you're just starting out—you won't.

A-LIST

A-list writers are the Hollywood screenwriting elite. They are highly paid, they have more favorable deals than other writers, and some are specialists in rewriting existing scripts rather than writing new stories.

ASSIGNMENT

Unlike a spec screenplay, which is the writer's original concept, an assignment script is for a project that has been developed in-house by a studio or producer. An assignment is often for an existing intellectual property—for example, the studio might own the rights to a novel and want it developed into a film. Writers often competitively pitch in order to be given access to these assignments.

BACK END

This refers to a profit-participation deal. You will get money "on the back end" if a movie does well.

BAKE-OFF

A modern phenomenon in which several writers compete against one another in rounds of pitching to be given an assignment. The bake-off, also known as "sweepstakes pitching," is a controversial business practice that may break **WGA** rules.

BEAT SHEET

A beat sheet usually refers to a short document outlining the key story moments in your script. You can glance at a beat sheet and understand the spine of the story, but it gives few details.

CONSIDER

A term used in **coverage**, in relationship to a writer or their script, that signifies possible interest or at least an acknowledgment that the work is promising or good.

COVERAGE

Before anyone important reads your script in an agency, studio, or producer's office, it will be read by a script reader who produces coverage. The reader's report becomes the basis for the institution's response to the script and will be read by executives before they decide whether it is worth their time to read the script itself. Coverage is archived by the company, so the chance that they will want to read your next script will depend in part on the coverage on your last one.

DEVELOPMENT

Development refers to the process in which a writer works with a producer or studio to take a **pitch** or **spec** all the way through to a **shooting script**. It may include the production of an **outline**, a **treatment**, a **beat sheet**, and other preparatory and persuasive documents, as well as a screenplay.

ELEVATOR PITCH

A short **pitch** that can be given quickly, as if you met an executive in an elevator and had until you reached the next floor to pitch your concept. This should last no more than 30 seconds.

GROSS POINTS

Profit participation in the gross profit of a movie. This can be very lucrative because you get paid before the accountants make the profit disappear.

HIGH CONCEPT

A movie idea that is easily communicated and has—or is deemed to have—wide appeal.

LOGLINE

A logline is an encapsulation of the concept of a screenplay in one sentence. The logline should tell you all you need to know to "get it."

MANAGER

Unlike many **agents**, managers take a more holistic view of their clients' career development and attempt to guide and nurture them. They are also more likely to be interested in emerging writers with potential. Unlike agents, managers do not negotiate contracts.

MBA

The Minimum Basic Agreement is the contract agreed between the **WGA** and the **AMPTP** every three years that sets out minimum compensation for writers working in Hollywood, and other terms like pension benefits and health coverage.

NET POINTS

Profit participation in the net profit of a movie. Given Hollywood accounting practices, you may never see money from net points.

ONE-STEP DEAL

A controversial modern deal under which the screenwriter is contracted to write a single draft of a screenplay. They may then be fired after submitting that draft. A typical studio deal used to guarantee one draft and one rewrite.

OUTLINE

An outline is a prosaic series of notes detailing the structure of a screenplay scene by scene. It is your plan, and it will keep you on track. Unlike **treatments**, outlines are documents used by writers more than executives.

PASS

A term used in **coverage** (and elsewhere) that means a rejection, as in: "We pass on your screenplay."

PITCH

A pitch is an oral presentation of your movie's concept. It should be short, pithy, and, like a **logline**, enable the listener to understand it right away. Although you should open with a very short statement—like a 30-second **elevator pitch**—that sells the concept, in a pitch meeting you will have a little more time to offer details about your story.

POLISH

A rewrite late in **development** that sometimes focuses on one aspect of the script, such as a "dialogue polish."

RECOMMEND

A term used very rarely in **coverage** to indicate work of the highest quality, or of particular interest to the producer, agency, or studio reviewing it.

RESIDUALS

These are royalties a writer gets when the movie or show they wrote is purchased on disc, screened, or streamed on television or in another market.

SHOOTING SCRIPT

A shooting script is a script that has gone through **development** and is ready to be filmed. It will have scene numbers attached and will follow well-established procedures in how revisions are incorporated (such as the use of colored paper).

SLUGLINE

In professional screenplay format, a slugline is the introductory statement that is inserted at the start of every scene. A slugline gives the reader information about the scene's location and time of day (or night). An example would be "INT. HOTEL—NIGHT", and so forth.

SPEC SCRIPT

A spec script is a screenplay written in the hope of a sale ("on spec" or speculatively), not as an assignment. Nobody asked for it, but hopefully they love it. It is probably what you intend to write with the help of this book.

SWEEPSTAKES PITCH-ING (SEE BAKE-OFF)

TREATMENT

A treatment is a persuasive document produced during **development** that tells the movie's story in prose. It doesn't go ploddingly through every single scene (that's an **outline**); rather, it sells the concept and key story moments. It is the first proof of concept—where the **pitch** was the concept—and may lead to a deal to write a screenplay. A very short treatment might be four pages; a very long treatment could be thirty pages.

WGA

The Writers Guild of America is the writers' union. There are two branches: Writers Guild of America, East, which is based in New York; and the Writers Guild of America West, in Los Angeles.

WRITERS' ROOM

This refers to the system in television production in which a group of writers and writer-producers work together, in the eponymous room, to break and develop stories for the show. *Saturday Night Live*, for example, has a famous writers' room.

"One of the things I like best about screenwriting: whatever is true, the opposite can also be true."

—Walter Hill, writer of *The Getaway* (1972) and *The Warriors* (1979)

KNOW THE MECHANICS

Screenwriting has a lot of rules, and there are good creative reasons to follow some standard practices and to resist others. Many of the great screenwriters bent, bypassed, or transcended the rules and, in so doing, changed the game for all of us. But first, you have to learn the rules.

In this chapter, we explore the basic mechanics of screenwriting. Here, "format" refers to everything from how the script's elements are laid out on the page to how writers describe events in a scene, and even the font and size of the letters they type. The rules of formatting are important to internalize and follow because they establish respect for your colleagues from every production department. It's also a way to signal your mastery of this creative endeavor on paper.

THE TWO FUNCTIONS OF A SCREENPLAY

To understand all this, we must remember that a screenplay serves two functions. First, it is a literary document. Your script is your story, and it should be compelling just like any good story, no matter its genre. Second, a screenplay is a shared technical document laying out a series of instructions that are used by everyone in development, production, and post-production. In addition to captivating future audiences with its content, your screenplay must communicate clearly and professionally. It directs the work of everyone whose name appears in the movie's credits.

Formatting is especially important for this second context because collaborators use your screenplay in different ways. They need to be able to easily find the information that is important *to them*. That information should be where they expect to find it. In other words: It should be formatted correctly into your screenplay.

Let's take the casting director on your movie. They certainly want to read your screenplay because they need to understand which performers might be a good fit for the project. But they need to find pieces of information quickly so that they can do their job efficiently. That's why the first time you introduce a character, you put their name in capital letters. The CAPS feature makes the name pop off the page and signals to your casting director there is a new role to cast. It's also important for the larger story to describe each character the first time you introduce them because, again, this is a literary document. Like much of screenwriting, formatting is both a creative and a functional task.

Every department will look at your script to find the information that is relevant to them. The director of photography looks for whether a scene is shot in the daytime or at night; the props team needs to know whether to bring an umbrella or a feather duster for the next day's shoot. Yet before we consider how to format a screenplay on the page in more detail, it's important to remember that even the length of your script comes under the rules of formatting.

FORMAT IS A GATEKEEPER

When you submit your screenplay to agents, managers, producers, studios, writing competitions, or festivals, the first thing a reader will notice is your format. Does your screenplay even look like a screenplay? If it doesn't, you will come across as an amateur and your script will probably not get read past page one or two. Format is a gatekeeper.

Nobody cares about the occasional formatting error as long as the script looks like a script. It's the same thing with grammar and spelling: A few typos won't sink your work, but a script that obviously hasn't been proofread will not pass muster.

That's why we are covering formatting as the first rule of screenwriting in this book. It's important for so many reasons, but now let's see how it actually works. There are six key standard elements to screenplay format and two lesser ones. We'll cover them one by one.

STANDARD LENGTHS

A feature screenplay is expected to fall within a standard range: 90 to 120 pages. There are minor variants—comedy often "plays faster," for example, and you get a little less screen time for your pages, but for a spec script, 90 to 120 is a good range. Assignment scripts—projects the studio develops in-house rather than buying—will vary and are often longer.

What is the general rule of thumb? A single screenplay page equates to one minute of screen time. Thus, a 90-page script equates to a 90-minute movie. It's not an exact science, of course, but the professional screenplay format has been developed over decades so that the match is pretty close. One reason feature films have historically conformed to this has to do with scheduling in cinemas. Frankly, it also had something to do with human bladders and our ability to resist restroom breaks!

Yet this expectation is changing in the era of streaming and big-budget tentpoles. When the audience is watching at home, the length is less of an issue. Tentpoles are expected to be longer. Have you seen a contemporary superhero movie shorter than two hours? Despite these market changes, for a spec script, 120 pages (or 120 minutes) should be your maximum. Nobody is going to care if your script is 122 pages, but if it creeps up to 125, 130, or higher, people will assume you don't know how to edit.

Incidentally, you might wonder why screenplays are still written in 12-point Courier, or "typewriter" font. It's because that font doesn't "kern" or adjust on the page, it is always a consistent size with consistent spacing. It is also about standardization: If everyone's using the same typeface, then everyone can be sure the page length formula is more or less correct.

How does page length translate into scenes? A rule of thumb is that a feature film contains somewhere around 60 to 65 scenes (nowadays more likely the latter), averaging about one and a half pages (minutes) each. This is much less set in stone than the page-length rule. The key takeaway here is that movie scenes tend to be short. A four-to-five-page scene is long, and most movies have only a few scenes of that length. You might, for example, save a longer scene for a major dramatic confrontation.

FORMATTING CHEAT SHEET

RULE: One script page = one minute of screen time
AVERAGE SPEC SCRIPT: 90 to 120 pages
AVERAGE NUMBER OF SCENES: 60 to 65 (~1.5 pages/minutes per scene)

MASTER SCENE FORMAT

First things first: Your screenplay should be written in *master scene format*. Master scene format is a way of writing scenes that describes action without specifically calling shots or camera direction. You describe the action in a scene as if you are looking at it in a master shot—a wide, long, or establishing lens that shows us everything that is going on. If this sounds abstract, it is. We'll dig into examples soon. The important thing is to describe the action as much as possible without directly naming shots (close-up, medium shot, etc.).

This is a major change from older formatting styles you may encounter if you read a screenplay from the classical Hollywood era. Before master scene format was adopted as the standard, screenplays were typically written as a list of shots. Nowadays, shooting scripts include more shot-calling and camera direction, but—for the most part—a spec screenplay should not. In reality, you may have to occasionally name shots when there is no efficient way of explaining what the audience will see in other terms, but you should avoid doing so whenever possible.

Here's a short, romantic example: It's the big date and Jane is going to tell Sophie that she loves her. In master scene format, you describe the interaction between the two of them as they walk hand in hand through the park at sunset, stare into each other's eyes, and then . . . Jane takes a deep breath and comes out with those three loaded words: "I love you." What will Sophie say? How will she react? It's a big deal for both of them and we can imagine how good acting and good directing will make this moment feel intense.

In a conventional movie, an important part of those creative choices will involve the director shooting coverage of the scene. "Coverage" in this sense is the list of shots the director will ask for to make sure that the scene can be edited properly in post-production, and that the drama of the scene will be effectively captured. Standard coverage would include some combination of medium shots, medium close-ups, over-the-shoulder shots, and close-ups of the two characters' dialogue and reactions. Maybe (cheese alert) there's a cutaway close-up of Jane taking Sophie's hand in hers.

The effect of the finished scene—the physical, emotional reaction we get from watching the film—comes from losing ourselves in those close-ups of the characters' reactions. But the screenplay doesn't call these shots. It just tells us what is happening and leaves the shot-calling for the director and the cinematographer to plan during their preparation for the shoot. That's the principle of master scene format. Now let's take a look at what actually goes on the page.

STANDARD ELEMENTS OF SCREENPLAY FORMAT

Remember: You write everything in `12-point Courier`.

Transition

The transition element is always in CAPS, positioned on the right-hand side of the page as a right indent. It informs the reader how we get from one scene to the next. Examples of common transitions include `CUT TO:` or `DISSOLVE TO:`. Transitions also start and finish a screenplay, typically with `FADE IN:` and `FADE TO BLACK:`, respectively.

Slugline or Scene Heading

You use a slugline or scene heading whenever you change location or time. Either change always prompts a transition to a new scene. That means scene B can be in the same space as scene A; only time has passed. Whenever you change scenes, you use a slugline.

The slugline contains three pieces of information, all written in CAPS:

1. Tell us whether the scene takes place inside or outside; interior or exterior, written as `INT.` or `EXT.` There are minor variations, such as `INT/EXT` when we follow a character as they run outside, or for scenes in vehicles.

2. Next, tell us where the scene is located: `JOE'S BASEMENT`, `THE JUNGLE`, `THE MAGICAL CITY OF BOB`.

3. Then, type a hyphen (in fact, space/hyphen/space), followed by the time: `DAY` or `NIGHT`. You can be more specific: `DAWN`, `DUSK`, and so forth. You can indicate that no time has passed since the previous scene (although the location has, because we are changing scenes) by writing `CONTINUOUS`. So, for example, you might use `CONTINUOUS` when characters

have been talking in a building (`INT.`) and then they walk out (`EXT.`) and we pick them up outside in the next scene, but as a continuous action.

Put it together and your slugline looks like this:

`INT. JOE'S BASEMENT - DAY`

Or:

`EXT. JUNGLE - NIGHT`

Or even:

`EXT. THE MAGICAL CITY OF BOB - CONTINUOUS`

Action (description)

The terms "action" and "description" are interchangeable, but I prefer "action" because it reminds me not to over-write. Under the slugline, use action to write what is happening in your scene. You'll write this in regular lowercase and using the entire width of the page. There is so much to be said about writing great action descriptions, but I'll give you a few quick tips here to get you started:

Indicate, but don't over-describe. Think of each sentence or moment under description as a kind of thought-image that works a bit like a shot without being explicitly called. When your simple description has done the basic job of helping us conjure up an image, then it's time to help us imagine the next one. Use a line of white space before describing the next moment in your scene. We will "see" your separated images in our minds like shots, even though you are not calling them.

Use white space to separate these thought-images. A screenplay page should not be a wall of text. Rather, it should make us want to skip over the white space to the next short, pithy piece of description.

First-time characters appear in all CAPS. Remember that when a character is introduced for the first time in the screenplay, their name should be in CAPS. Include a brief line or two of description, including their age (usually in parentheses). Here's how Tom Cruise's character Ray is described in the first scene of *War of the Worlds* (2005):

```
RAY (in his 30s, short hair, rough
groomed, almost always wears his New York
baseball cap, raggedly dressed, looks
like he hasn't slept in days)...;
```

(Note: You usually wouldn't put the whole description in parenthesis, just the age.)

Make your writing as kinetic as the action that will replace it on the screen. Sometimes, especially when writing an action sequence—a fight, a chase, a sporting event, etc.—grammar will take a back seat to the dynamic use of language. There are many ways to do this, but one simple option is to split sentences and use ellipses or hyphenation to draw the reader from image to image, moment to moment. Here's a short example from *Terminator Salvation* (2009), written by John Brancato & Michael Ferris:

```
It SNAPS its ELONGATED TEETH at him, but
he manages to BREAK its neck and hurl
it toward --

TWO MORE SKINDOGS moving in for an attack.
```

SAGE SPOTLIGHT:
THE PRINCESS BRIDE

Screenwriters can engage their readers in the moment by throwing out the rules of grammar and syntax, becoming creative with page layout. This example is from William Goldman's screenplay for *The Princess Bride* (1987).

```
                                    CUT TO:

THE DARKNESS BEHIND THEM

And there's still nothing to be
seen. It's still ominous.

Only now it's eerie too.

Then --

The moon slips through and --

Inigo was right -- something is
very much there. A sailboat. Black.
With a great billowing sail. Black.
It's a good distance behind them,
but it's coming like hell, closing
the gap.
```

When writing action, ask yourself two questions:

1. How long will the events you are describing on the page take to play out on-screen? Does it earn its page space in those terms? Remember, half a page is 30 seconds.

2. Can you afford all the words you just wrote? Remember: You only have a maximum of 120 script pages. The longer your action descriptions are, the fewer scenes you get to write.

It's a tricky balance. Sometimes a longer description sells the drama or the spectacle in a way that totally justifies its length. My advice is to save space for those crucial moments and cut back elsewhere when you can.

Note: Did you notice the ampersand in the writers' credit for *Terminator Salvation* on page 21? When two or more writers are linked with an ampersand on a screenplay or in movie credits, it means they wrote together as a team. When they are linked with "and" it means they wrote separate drafts.

Character Name

The next format element introduces who is speaking dialogue. The name of the speaker is in CAPS, centered on the page with a line of its own, thus:

```
                    INES
```

Parenthetical

Sometimes the dialogue a character is speaking needs explanation or qualification, particularly if they are speaking in a language other than English. That's when you use a parenthetical. This format element either comes between the character name and the dialogue or is inserted between lines of dialogue. Thus:

```
                    INES
                (in Spanish)
```

Dialogue

Format the character's dialogue in a column running down the center of the page. Note that in this example the character is speaking Spanish, but the dialogue is written in English so that English-speaking readers can understand it. It probably doesn't matter for a simple and familiar statement, but for more complex dialogue you should always write in the primary language of your potential industry readers, thus:

```
                    INES
                (in Spanish)
     Good evening and welcome to my party.
     I hope you all enjoy yourselves tonight.
```

Splitting the dialogue with a parenthetical works like this:

```
                    INES
                (in Spanish)
     Good evening and welcome to my party.
                (in English)
     I hope you all enjoy yourselves tonight.
```

Extension

Less an element than an addendum to an element, an extension is placed after a character name (but before dialogue) to indicate when a character is off-screen or otherwise not present in the shot. For example, `INES(O.S.)` means she is off-screen and `INES(V.O.)` means we hear her as a voice-over, not merely speaking while she is out of frame. Remember to use CAPS for the entire line.

Shot

Now, strictly speaking, this element is a rule-breaker for the master scene format, but you'll likely come across it in some form or other. There are a number of ways in which calling a shot is acceptable in a screenplay. The important thing is not to overdo it and clutter up your script.

A simple example is when you need us to "see" an insert—something hidden or a detail. Some writers use a statement like CLOSE ON, aligned to the left of the page after a line of white space, to signify a cutaway, thus:

```
CLOSE ON: The tiny TRACKING DEVICE in
Jim's outstretched palm.
```

Most called shots in a master scene are situational. A good format book like Christopher Riley's *The Hollywood Standard* will give you a number of useful options. (See details in the Additional Resources section at the back of the book.)

Hand Props

You may have noticed the use of CAPS to draw attention to an important hand prop above. That's a common way of drawing the attention of the prop department. This works just like the rule that puts the first appearance of every character in CAPS. People need to use your screenplay to find information quickly, and CAPS pull the eye. Some people capitalize practical special effects that will happen in front of the camera (GRAVEL SPRAYS as bullets hit the ground), as opposed to digital special effects that happen in post-production.

GENERAL BEST PRACTICES

Here are some basic principles of formatting and technical screenwriting to bear in mind:

Less is almost always more. Give your readers just enough information to get the picture. We don't need every detail.

Avoid formatting "ticks." For example, many screenwriters use the word "beat" as a shorthand to indicate a small pause in action or dialogue. Bad writers use "beat" every other line. It gets annoying to read very fast. Sparingly please.

Don't put information where it shouldn't be. Use formatting elements for their intended purpose. The biggest culprit here is the overuse of action placed in the parenthetical. Unless you're *Princess Bride* screenwriter William Goldman, you're not allowed to do this, and I know you're not William Goldman because he's dead.

Don't over-direct character reactions. Let your drama and dialogue speak for themselves. Actors and directors hate when you micromanage them. A page of dialogue with no action description is fine.

Don't be redundant. If we can see something happening on-screen because you have already described it, don't have characters talk about what we can see.

The old maxim: Show, don't tell. Film is a visual medium, so try and communicate visually as much as possible. Don't be frightened of leaving things verbally unsaid.

Tell us what they do and say. Finally, and this is a big one: We can't read people's minds, so don't *tell* us what a character is thinking in your ACTION description. Tell us what they *do*. Tell us what they *say*. If your scene is any good, we can infer the rest.

In the Writers' Room:
FORMATTING EXERCISE

FORMAT THIS SCENE:

A family is gathered for dinner in their home. They join hands for the father to say grace, but the son is looking slyly down at his lap, waiting for his girlfriend to text him on his cell phone.

USE THE FOLLOWING:

1. A SLUGLINE, with location and time.
2. A line or two of ACTION that tells us what is going on. (Specify characters that are present but assume we have seen them before so there is no need to describe them in detail.)
3. A CHARACTER element, to introduce FATHER as the speaker.
4. A DIALOGUE element, as he says grace.
5. A SHOT direction, revealing the hidden cell phone on the son's lap.
6. A TRANSITION, to send us to the next scene.

Question: How will you communicate the son's *intention* when we can't read his mind? Show, don't tell.

UNDERSTAND STORY STRUCTURE

We can't talk about screenwriting without at least considering the three-act paradigm. It is likely you've heard this term, even if you are just starting out as a screenwriter. Whether or not you choose to adhere to it, it's important that you know what it means and how it is used.

From the early 1980s, the three-act paradigm became the default language of Hollywood development. This means that many, but not all, movie executives have been trained to think in terms of, and expect you to write in, three acts. This will impact the way you think about your own mode of storytelling and will thereby shape your outline, and (where appropriate) your treatment.

Not all Hollywood movies conform to the three-act paradigm. However, if you are working for a studio or major independent, you need to at least be able to think and speak to these terms—even when you plan to break the rules.

THE DISTINGUISHED THREE-ACT PARADIGM

The three-act paradigm is a model of storytelling that divides your screenplay into three big logical segments, or units of drama, each of which achieves a specific task. We generally think of these segments as beginning, middle, and end—or exposition, confrontation, and resolution. There are many ways to innovate from here; for example a character-centered version could be broken into exposition, character change, and resolution. The structure has a rich tradition in human storytelling. Let's take a deeper look.

Why Three Acts?

The historical answer is Aristotle. In his treatise *Poetics*, from around 335 BCE, the Greek philosopher established a model for writing tragedy. There, he defined three key storytelling elements: the beginning, the middle, and the end. Aristotle also divided the structure of tragedies into two segments: complication and unravelling (very loosely, the set-up and resolution), so his model isn't the simple match to three acts that some writers believe it is. Nevertheless, *Poetics* is incredibly influential in the history of dramatic writing.

Fast-forward to Hollywood, and the movie industry answer is Syd Field. The screenwriting legend popularized the term in his influential 1979 book *Screenplay*. Field was the guy who boiled story down and made it make sense to non-screenwriters. Many how-to books came after (like this one), but it was through *Screenplay* that modern Hollywood cemented its vocabulary around the three-act paradigm.

Does It Work?

Robert McKee explains in his book *Story* that the three-act structure is a set of principles that has emerged over time. It can be a remarkably flexible way of taming wild words and containing the causal logic of a story. Notably, it is used successfully across mediums. The three-act paradigm has been particularly effective in genre movies in which formulas play an even bigger role.

The three-act paradigm isn't a simple, reductive formula, although its relative ubiquity has drawn that accusation. Another critique is that the three-act structure is great if you want to tell an unrealistic moral fable in which everything happens for a reason and the ending ties things up in a neat bow. Real life isn't like that, critics argue.

Once you start reading screenwriting literature, you will encounter many variations of the three-act paradigm. The first thing to be aware of is that most of them are functionally the same. What they give you is different-size story bites to chew on.

Ultimately, it's up to you whether you want to follow the tried-and-true model or break form entirely. The important thing is that you are intentional not only about the story you want to tell, but also how you want to tell it. This is what structure is all about.

A Three-Act Story in Action: *Winter's Bone*

Adapting *Winter's Bone* (2010) for the screen, Debra Granik & Anne Rosellini used the closed-mouthed criminal culture of the Missouri Ozarks to add naturalism and believability to a three-act structure. In this film, the act structure is pretty conventional. In act one, Ree Dolly, a poor Missouri teenager who looks after her younger siblings as her mother deals with mental illness, finds out that her dad put the family's house and land up as collateral for bail before he disappeared. She sets out to find him, but nobody will help.

In act two she persists, despite being warned off. Her uncle, Teardrop, begins to take an interest and gradually becomes committed to helping her. At the midpoint, having learned that her father failed to show up at court—and that she has a week to find him or their home will be forfeit—Ree publicly calls out Thump Milton, head of their meth-cooking clan.

In response, women in Thump's circle beat Ree badly. They consider killing her, but Teardrop arrives and says he will take responsibility for Ree. Everyone is scared of Teardrop. Ree and Teardrop keep searching but can't find anything. It becomes clear that Ree's dad is likely dead because he began to talk to the sheriff. Teardrop angers dangerous locals as they hunt for him.

In act three, the disruption Ree has been making pays off when the women who beat her arrive to take her to her dad's body. They cut off his hands with a chainsaw and Ree delivers them to the authorities as evidence that he is dead.

At the end, the house is saved and Ree is given some money that was left from her dad's bail. At the same time, Teardrop tells her that he knows who killed her dad. Thus, the movie ends with Ree's immediate problem solved, but with Teardrop about to respond—and probably die—in the ensuing blood feud.

The most unconventional thing about *Winter's Bone* is the pacing of its causality. Granik and Rosellini sometimes delay showing the effects of Ree's attempts to get help and support, leaving her apparently stymied. When help comes, it seems like there is no immediate cause, but, of course, change happens slowly in this world. It takes time for a "no" to become a "yes." Spending time with Ree when it looks like she is defeated and friendless also binds us to her emotionally. In the end, Ree is the architect of her family's salvation over three acts, but the writers play the movie's conventional structure to the pace and rhythm of its story world, not to those of tentpole Hollywood.

IS THE THREE-ACT PARADIGM RIGHT FOR ME?

Here's a list of issues that will help you decide if the three-act paradigm is going to be the structural model best suited for your story. If the answer to most of these questions is "yes," then the three-act paradigm is probably a good fit for you.

1. Is your story in a popular genre (horror, science fiction, rom-com, thriller, etc.)?
2. Is your protagonist strongly goal driven?
3. Is your story concept plot driven?
4. Do you want the ending of your story to tie everything up neatly?
5. Is this a story that involves major character change for your protagonist?
6. Is this story aimed squarely at mainstream Hollywood?

If you answered mostly "no" to these questions, then you might want to think twice about using a straightforward three-act paradigm and consider other options, maybe pushing the boundaries even further than we saw with the alternate causality pacing in the example of *Winter's Bone*.

BREAKOUT STAR:
Ava DuVernay on Committing to Be a Screenwriter

Screenwriter, director, producer, and distributor Ava DuVernay worked as a publicist for more than a decade before she wrote and directed her first microbudget short film. Since releasing the film in 2006, she's become a critical darling and an Emmy, BAFTA, and Peabody Award winner. The director of *Selma* (2014) and *A Wrinkle in Time* (2018) and the writer-director of the Oscar-nominated documentary *13th* (2016) talked to Scott Meyers at the Black List about the process of becoming a writer:

"For so long I felt like, 'I'm never going to be able to be a screen-writer, because I have this other job, or I have this other thing that I'm doing to make a living.' Really, my lesson was—and it's helped me in a lot of other ways—that to do something, to be something, you don't have to be all-in right away. Writing at night, writing on the weekends, dipping your toe into something is okay! You go on a hike and you explore, doesn't mean you have to build a house there. You're just going and walking around. Do that with your dreams. I think that for me if there's any lesson, especially for folks that are looking to maybe switch from one career to another, or to dip their toe in directing, writing, or filmmaking, is that it's not all or nothing. That you can explore, that you can figure out if it works for you, that you can take risks that are not as risky. You don't need to walk away from your life in order to follow your dream right away. That was something that was a big, big lesson. For so long, I felt really trapped in publicity, or 'This is my job,' or 'I can't risk not having my health insurance,' or 'How am I going to live?' My mind immediately went to an all-or-nothing scenario to pursue a dream. It doesn't necessarily have to be that way. You can dream a bit at a time."

STRUCTURAL OUTLIERS

Not every movie follows the three-act paradigm. In this section, we'll look at some alternative ways of telling your story. The outliers here are in the minority, but they are also some of the most memorable instances of cinematic storytelling in independent cinema in recent decades. When diverging from the norm works, it often works powerfully.

Non-Chronological Plots

Sometimes non-chronological plots use repeated flashback structures to reveal truth and establish motivation. This is the case in Quentin Tarantino's *Reservoir Dogs* (1992), when we come to understand that Mr. Orange is an undercover cop. Other times, these types of plots present events out of sequence as a way of evoking the workings of memory, like in Scott Neustadter and Michael H. Weber's *500 Days of Summer* (2009), or to emphasize theme in some other way.

Another iteration of the non-chronological plot is a circular narrative, like in Tarantino's *Pulp Fiction* (1994), where story elements are presented out of order to allow their symbolic and thematic interplay to work on the audience as a kind of genre treat. David Lynch and Barry Gifford's neo-noir *Lost Highway* (1997) uses circularity to establish and (possibly) resolve a psychological puzzle about the nature of the protagonist. While a chronological structure is the right choice for most screenplays, a well-executed non-chronological structure can be the key to making a movie work.

Multi-Plot Structures

Multi-plot movies typically divide their story time between different character groups whose activities are discreet but also relate to the movie's overarching plot and theme. Multi-plot movies are distinct from ensembles in part because there are fewer subplots and characters involved. An example is *Much Ado About Nothing* (1993), in which separate love plots intertwine. Another is *Contagion* (2011), which shows us a pandemic unfolding from a range of perspectives.

There is also the anthology film, such as *Sin City* (2005), which follows a range of characters in intertwining hard-boiled stories, and *Mystery Train* (1989), which combines three short stories about people from different countries in Memphis, Tennessee. Other anthologies simply collect short works by different filmmakers around a central concept or theme. A multi-plot structure encourages the audience to focus on big themes or concepts rather than individuals.

Ensemble-Led Structures

There are two typical forms of ensemble-led story structure. The first, and most common, has a defined lead, or leads, but gives other characters their own threads, subplots, or times to shine. *Ocean's 8* (2018) and *The Dirty Dozen* (1967) would be examples of this story type.

The other common ensemble structure gives us a number of characters who have independent plot arcs, but their actions are connected thematically. Good recent examples of this would be *Love Actually* (2003), in which a number of couples, and prospective couples, explore love from different perspectives. In a much more thematically complex fashion, screenwriter Guillermo Arriaga weaves together four stories that are linked by one thoughtless violent incident in *Babel* (2006).

Minimal Plot

Some people use the term "non-causal," but I prefer to think of minimal plot movies, where there is always some causal path one can take in watching them. This includes films where something other than conventional plotting sustains our engagement, such as when style or the interaction of mannered characters takes precedence over plot. In movies of this kind, we follow the actions of characters who don't do much, and that's the point.

One example of a minimal plot is Jim Jarmusch's long-take movie *Stranger Than Paradise* (1984), where we follow two bored gamblers and a visiting cousin from Hungary as they hang out in New York City (act one), Cleveland (act two), and Florida (act three). Not a lot happens, but the minimalist cinematic structure underpins the characters' languid interactions. This structure—defined by a lack of clear structure—is extremely hard to execute well.

ACTS AND BEATS

We started with a story divided into three acts. From here we can further divide into sequences, or *beats*, each of which significantly advances the story. Here we'll look at a story structure with nine beats, which can play in different lengths, depending on how you want them to affect your audience. A story beat can land on a single image or line of dialogue, or it can take twenty minutes to play out.

In this way, each movie story will likely place different emphasis on individual beats depending on the story's genre, style, goal, and theme. Often, but not always, the longer beats are the ones where the story needs more narrative weight to make its case. Conversely, short beats are usually very clear and purposeful, not requiring subtle development.

At least in broad strokes, the format presented below works for any narrative film you want to write, short of the truly experimental. We are going to work this through using the structure of *Jojo Rabbit* (2019), which won its writer/director, Taika Waititi, the Oscar for Best Adapted Screenplay (from the novel *Caging Skies*, by Christine Leunens) as a case study.

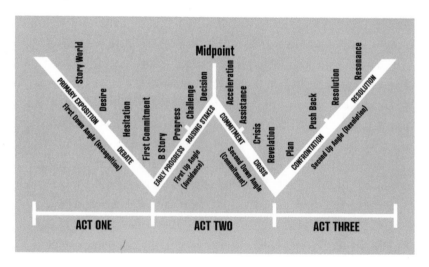

Act One Beats

Act one is relatively short in most feature films, probably lasting under 30 minutes for a 90-minute movie. It establishes your protagonist in their world and sets up the goal or theme of your story. At the end of act one, your protagonist has decided, however reluctantly, to try and achieve their goal and resolve their theme. Here are the two big beats.

Primary Exposition

The movie begins in a world in which your protagonist has a problem or a desire. We see what they lack. Soon an event focuses their mind on that goal or overlays it with a bigger problem. This is your inciting incident.

An inciting incident is the event that gets the story moving. In the first act of a conventional Hollywood movie we meet our protagonist(s) and learn about their goals and dreams. Then, something dramatic happens to derail them or to set them on the road to achieving those dreams (or failing to achieve them, bravely or amusingly). In a romantic comedy, the star-crossed lovers meet. In a slasher movie, the killer is activated. In a revenge movie, somebody hurts your protagonist, or the people they love.

Knowing your movie's inciting incident is very useful because it immediately gives your concept personal stakes. It evokes your protagonist's own desire or need and thus brings the rest of the story or plot into focus. (We'll go into deeper detail on the inciting incident in rule 3; for now, let's focus on how it plays into the overall structure.)

In *Jojo Rabbit*, this beat lands fast and hard as we watch ten-year-old Jojo putting on his Hitler Youth uniform. This is followed by a reveal where we learn that Jojo has a weirdly comical version of Adolf Hitler as his imaginary friend. Jojo swears he will devote all his strength to Hitler.

Jojo is fanatically keen to do well at an upcoming camp excursion for young Nazis. He can't wait to prove himself and become a man. This establishes growing up as the main theme of the movie.

In the inciting incident, Jojo is ordered to kill a rabbit to prove his courage and manhood. He refuses, and the other members of the Hitler Youth bully him for being a coward, calling him "Jojo Rabbit."

Debate

Your protagonist really wants the thing—or to avoid the thing—but they don't know how to get it, or whether they can. The thing the protagonist wants will relate directly to the story's theme.

At the end of act one, we have established what and who the story is about. Your protagonist has also *debated* whether and how to try and achieve their goal. They have made a first commitment to do so, but it is weak, contingent, or unrealistic. Now they need to get their act together, and that's what act two is all about.

In *Jojo Rabbit*, the debate beat is short. After refusing to kill the rabbit, Jojo's imaginary Hitler friend appears and cheers him up, persuading him that rabbits are brave, too. "Be the rabbit," imaginary Hitler tells him. "Be brave and sneaky and strong." Encouraged, Jojo rushes back to where his fellow kids are practicing throwing live grenades. Full of enthusiasm to prove himself, Jojo makes a first commitment to being brave and strong (to growing up). Running forward, he throws a grenade, which bounces back off a tree and explodes at his feet, injuring his face and leg. He is taken to the hospital.

Remember that first commitment beats at the end of act one are about showing how far the protagonist still has to go to achieve what they seek. The accident with the grenade does just that.

Act Two Beats

Act two takes your protagonist from being willing but incapable of achieving their goals to having a real chance of doing so. That means second acts are all about character change. In a plot-driven movie, change can also mean getting the thing that will help you win—a powerful weapon, a big clue, an ally, a plan, or all of the above.

Act two is usually the longest act in your movie, roughly 45 minutes for a 90-minute film, and we can split it into two sections. The first leads up to the midpoint, which is a second key decision point for your protagonist. At the midpoint, they make another commitment to achieve their goals, only this time they know that after making their choice, there will be no going back. Midpoint commitments are typically courageous, so they often transform protagonists into heroes or heroines.

After the midpoint, everything accelerates and gets much harder. Your protagonist is tested to their limit as they learn how to achieve their goals.

Early Progress

Your protagonist starts working toward their goal. At first it is easy; they make some progress. Soon the antagonistic forces begin to gather and push back.

Jojo is on the mend, but he feels useless. Two significant events happen: First, Jojo sees the bodies of executed traitors hanging in the main square, which jarringly reveals the dark side of the Nazi regime. Second, Jojo discovers that there is a young Jewish woman named Elsa who is hiding, with his mother's knowledge, in a crawl space in their home.

Elsa threatens him that if he reveals her presence, he and his mother will be punished. They begin a strange series of interactions where Jojo interrogates her and wants to learn more about Jews. He starts by referring to racist stereotypes, and she responds mockingly. They gradually learn more about one another, and Jojo's questions become more rational and insightful.

Raising Stakes

Making progress becomes harder and harder. Now your protagonist has to make a second commitment. This time they know the stakes. This time there will be no going back.

In *Jojo Rabbit*, Jojo argues with his mother, blaming her for many things. On the one hand he is angry with her for hiding a Jew. On the other, he is becoming fonder of Elsa as he gets to know her. The contradictory pressures in the house are increasing and Jojo's emotional connection to Elsa is bringing him closer to rejecting the lies he has been taught by the outside world.

We also infer that Jojo's mother is working against the Nazis in other ways, although the details are not made clear.

Midpoint

Your protagonist makes that second commitment. Good for them. Maybe they just became a hero.

The midpoint in *Jojo Rabbit* is subtle, but emotionally eloquent. It also happens after the halfway point in terms of running time, because the story places its emphasis on Jojo's slow learning curve in humanizing his view of Elsa and, through her, Jewish people in general. This process is given a lot of screen time and the payoff, when it comes at the midpoint, feels earned because of it.

Having been told by his mother that he'll know he is in love when he gets butterflies in his stomach, Jojo experiences this feeling for Elsa. His interiority is represented on screen by a literal superimposition of a cluster of butterflies in his stomach. After this moment, there is no doubt that Jojo is turning away from his Nazi obsession and toward humanity and emotional maturity.

Love is his second commitment and it is immediately tested in the commitment beat when the Gestapo turn up.

Commitment

Immediately the stakes are raised, and the pushback gets fierce. Fortunately, there is usually some form of assistance available from friends and allies made along the way.

In *Jojo Rabbit*, the Gestapo search Jojo's house, raising the stakes immediately. Elsa pretends to be Jojo's dead sister, Inge, and Jojo plays along—see how he has changed already? Captain Klenzendorf, who works with the Hitler Youth and has taken a liking to Jojo, helps verify Elsa/Inge's identity and the Gestapo leave.

Crisis

Your protagonist is beaten down (emotionally or physically) to their lowest point by the antagonistic forces in your story. This is their crisis. Here they are at their lowest. However, seeing and experiencing things as they truly are, and with the help of the allies they have made along the way, your protagonist sees the way forward. The odds are long, but at least they have a plan. Putting that plan into action is what act three is all about.

In *Jojo Rabbit*, Jojo goes into the main square to find that his mother has been hanged as a traitor. In his grief and rage, he attacks Elsa.

Imaginary Hitler tries to persuade him to get with the Nazi program, but Jojo isn't convinced.

Jojo and Elsa then have a real heart-to-heart for the first time. She tells him what she knows of his parents, treating him as an equal, because he has earned it through his emotional pain.

Act Three Beats

Act three is also relatively short, coming in at under 30 minutes. It is probably the shortest act of all in most movies. It is all about your prepared protagonist enacting their plan to achieve their goals and to resolve their theme. There will be a final test and then (usually) success. We leave your story contemplating the protagonist's world as it has been changed by the resolution. Here are the two big beats.

Confrontation

The plan made at the end of act two gets put into action. With every plan there is pushback: The antagonistic forces make a final stand.

In *Jojo Rabbit*, external forces put pressure on Jojo and Elsa. He searches for food in the rubble of the city. Occupation is near, but will it be the Americans or the Soviets? The final battle is imminent.

Jojo is caught up in the chaos of the fighting. Germany is defeated and the US and Soviet occupiers take over. Jojo, who is wearing a German army shirt, is nearly executed by Russian soldiers, but Captain Klenzendorf saves him by pretending Jojo is a Jew and spitting on him. Jojo lives, while Captain Klenzendorf is shot.

Resolution

Success! Or dramatically satisfying failure! The goal is achieved. The theme is resolved. The world, and the protagonist, have been changed by the story. Let us see that change before the movie ends.

In *Jojo Rabbit*, Jojo delays telling Elsa that it is safe to come out of hiding because he doesn't want her to leave. In the end, he shows how much he has grown and tells Elsa he loves her, understanding that she can't love him back in that way. He leads her outside and they dance together in happiness.

THE ROLE OF CONFLICT

In terms of structure, a story becomes dramatic (drama = conflict) when your protagonist encounters opposition to their goals. We see conflict implied or specified in many of the beats in *Jojo Rabbit's* structure.

Ideally, your protagonist and their opponents—including the story's antagonist(s)—should have goals that are linked to your story's theme. If you populate your story with characters who have different takes, attitudes, needs, and desires in relationship to the same theme, then their interactions—their conflict—becomes especially vital and dramatic.

In *Despicable Me* (2010), the protagonist, Gru, wants to be the world's greatest villain. His antagonist, Vector, shares the same goal. That brings them into conflict in the plot, and that plot conflict helps to expose and explore Gru's inner motivations in the story. In *How to Train Your Dragon* (2010), the antagonist, Stoick the Vast, wants to deal with the problem of marauding dragons, as does his teenage son, the protagonist, Hiccup. They just have different takes on how to do so. In the film, Hiccup understands the dragons and wants to make friends. Stoick doesn't understand the creatures and wants to wipe them out, hence the family conflict. This example reminds us of an important principle: An antagonist doesn't have to be evil. Antagonists simply embody or represent oppositional forces to your protagonist; there is no necessary moral component to what they do.

And some opponents have very simple goals with no moral aspect. The wolf pack is hungry and your protagonist smells like lunch. The wolves may not have complex characterization. But in a wilderness movie, where survival is the theme and the antagonist *is* the wilderness, then simple opponents play out your theme.

How do we use conflict in a movie script? Screenwriters use conflict in many ways, but two of the most important are to raise stakes and to test character.

Raising the Stakes

In *Star Wars: Episode IV - A New Hope*, Han Solo says, "Good against remotes is one thing. Good against the living? That's something else."

Han speaks for many screenwriters in anticipating that things are going to get much harder in the future. Raising stakes is fun. It proves that your antagonist is a true challenge, that your obstacles are major obstacles, and that nobody gets things easy in a good story. Here are a couple of examples of how it can work:

1. Hungry wolves chase your protagonist, Lily, into a cave. There's a bear in the cave. It's a mama bear, and Lily just tripped over her cub in the dark. The stakes are officially raised.

2. Your protagonist, Jen, meets up with her ex Kelly, hoping to rekindle the romance. But now Kelly's dating another ex, Alex. And Alex really hates Jen. Oh, and by the way, the next morning at work, guess who just got head-hunted and is Jen's new line manager? Yup, it's Alex. Stakes officially raised.

Raising stakes overlaps with the second key use of conflict in a screenplay: We raise the stakes to test our characters.

Testing Character, i.e., Creating Obstacles

Conflict makes your protagonist work hard. Conflict that is targeted at their weaknesses, or insecurities, makes them work even harder. If Lily can get out of the wolf/bear sandwich alive, she'll have proved something. If Jen can untangle her work/dating mess, she'll have proved something. In these cases, we've tested our characters by creating meaningful obstacles.

In *How to Train Your Dragon*, there is also a gigantic dragon queen who must be defeated in order for the other dragons to be free. This dragon is certainly the most dangerous enemy in the movie, but she's not the antagonist because she doesn't represent the movie's theme. Stoick is the antagonist; the dragon queen is an obstacle.

When the dragon queen attacks the clan's warriors, all appears to be lost. Then Hiccup rides his friendly dragon to the rescue, leading the other teenagers mounted on their own dragons. Stoick finally understands he was wrong about dragons, and wrong about his son. The theme of the movie resolves at his apology to Hiccup, but there's still a giant dragon to defeat. Once again: obstacle, not antagonist.

Obstacles are a test of character, whether emotionally, physically, or intellectually, and they show us how far your protagonist has come on their path to achieving their goals and resolving their theme.

In the Writers' Room:
PLOT EXERCISE

This exercise is about how characters generate conflict and, thus, story and plot. It starts from the simple proposition that opinions make people angry. Indeed, they cause conflict. Your protagonist is opinionated. She always has a view on everything, big issue or small.

1. For this exercise, I want you to pick six issues about which your protagonist has a strong opinion. They don't all have to be about religion or politics, although they can be of course. She could be, for example, an atheist and a libertarian. Those are big, life-defining issues, and yet she also has definite ideas about small things, like the best way to cook lasagna, or which actor was the best James Bond (it was Sean Connery, fight me).

   Remember that the surface opinions someone holds likely imply deeper emotional, intellectual, or other psychological work that is going on in their psyche. Are they an atheist because their parents were also, or because their parents were evangelicals and they are rebelling, or because they have studied and considered issues of faith and science deeply? Why might a character care deeply about lasagna recipes? It could have something to do with their ethnicity, immigrant status, class allegiance, desire to travel, search for some kind of authenticity in their own life, a need for structure, or deep emotional ties to unresolved childhood issues. If you dig deep

CONTINUED ►

    enough, you can wrap a movie around a love of early Bond movies . . .

2. Now invent four other characters and establish their basic relationships with your protagonist, be they friends, relatives, romantic partners, ex-lovers, work colleagues, or whatever.

3. Now give them all personal attitudes to each of your protagonist's opinions.

4. Now ask yourself: How does your population of opinionated characters lead to a theme (discussed in detail in rule 3), to conflict, and to a plot?

DEVELOP YOUR STORY

Now that you understand a bit more about story structure, we are going to develop that story, digging deeper into the theme that drives your story and its subplots. Our initial point of focus will be the inciting incident in your first act.

This catalytic moment—this call to action—is an essential marker that helps integrate your theme into your story and plot. There are different types of inciting incidents, but what unites them all is the work they make the protagonist do in facing their hopes, their dreams, and their failings.

From here, we'll go through the building blocks you'll need for your story, focusing on how characters drive plot arcs and how stories are logical constructions built upon themes. Then, we'll discuss how to tie everything together.

START WITH THE INCITING INCIDENT

A quick reminder that an inciting incident is an occurrence early in the movie's plot that puts the whole story into motion. Before the inciting incident, the world of the protagonist is typically in stasis. They may be doing well but going nowhere; they might be in dire need, materially or emotionally. They might be ready for change, even if they don't know it yet. The story is going to test them, whether they like it or not. The inciting incident will get things going. In general, there are two primary types of inciting incidents: character-driven and "coincidental." Let's have a look.

Character-Driven Inciting Incidents

Character-driven inciting incidents emerge from your protagonist or their interaction with other characters. Your protagonist might realize they have to do something, or someone else might persuade them to do something to change or improve their life. This kind of inciting incident encourages your protagonist to make an active and purposeful choice.

In *Parasite* (2019), co-written by Bong Joon Ho and Han Jin Won, the role of protagonist is actually shared between members of the financially struggling Kim family. Near the start, a friend (Min Hyuk) suggests to the son, Kim Ki Woo, that he take over tutoring a wealthy girl for him while he travels abroad. From this simple suggestion, Ki Woo's entire family gets involved in working for and deceiving the wealthy family. The plot develops, or rather spirals out, from here. In this case, the inciting incident is driven by character, because Min Hyuk knows Ki Woo needs the money and that he is capable of doing the job. He's doing his friend a favor.

In the opening sequence of *The World's End* (2013), Gary tells the story of the epic, although never-completed, pub crawl he went on with his friends after they left school. He admits that was the best night of his life. We cut to middle-aged Gary, a loser in an AA meeting, and it is revealed that he has been telling this story to the group. Somebody asks him if he ever wished he had finished the pub crawl—if he wishes he had made it to The World's End, the last pub on the list. Gary says no, but we track in on his face as the idea hits. He's going to get the old gang back together and finish the pub crawl, because that'll solve everything, right?

Coincidental Inciting Incidents

In the case of coincidental inciting incidents, our protagonist is getting on with their life and then something extraordinary happens. The incident itself isn't linked to them, but the choices they will have to make in order to deal with it still speak to the core of their problems and desires.

In the opening of *North by Northwest* (1959), the Alfred Hitchcock thriller written by Ernest Lehman, advertising executive Roger Thornhill is mistaken for another man. This minor incident starts Roger down a trail toward danger and adventure as he becomes the focus and victim of the other man's enemies. Thornhill is a victim of coincidence, simply in the wrong place at the wrong time, and that's how Hitchcock likes it.

There is a subset of these categories that we might call mysterious or ambivalent inciting incidents. In these cases, the motivation for the incident is unclear or interpreted one way by the audience. When it occurs, we are waiting for the real truth to be discovered, whether we know it or not. These ambivalent inciting incidents still tend to resolve toward the character-driven or the coincidental. Here's a good example: In *Alien* (1979), the crew is woken up because they are told the ship has received a distress signal and they are obliged to investigate. They board the derelict spacecraft. Later in the story, the crew works out that the signal may have been a warning. Later still, Warrant Officer Ripley finds out that the ship was rerouted specifically to investigate a life form—the alien of the title—and to gather a specimen. So, to begin with, we assume the inciting incident is coincidental; the ship just happened to receive the signal, and off they go. As the story develops, we learn the inciting incident was triggered so that Ash (the science officer) would take action to preserve the alien.

As you can see from these examples, the inciting incident prompts your goal-driven protagonist toward action. That action is expressed in the story, in the plot, and through relationships with other characters.

No Incident, Smooth Sailing?

If there really is no causality in your movie at all, well, that's outside the scope of this book. You're an experimental filmmaker, and I look forward to seeing your work: live your truth. But pretty much every movie that comes within sniffing distance of a narrative has an inciting incident of some kind. Some of them are very low-key, but in the end, no matter how you define "story" in your movie, it has to start and end somehow.

You don't have to have aliens land in your backyard or have your protagonist see the person of their dreams walk past in cheesy slow motion. But where there is no beginning, there is no movie. As a general rule of thumb: If there is causality of any kind in your movie, then there has to be a first cause.

Sometimes an unconventional inciting incident may even happen off-screen or before the movie starts. In the Duplass brothers' micro-budget road movie *The Puffy Chair* (2005), Josh sees an ad for a chair that reminds him of one his dad used to have. He decides to buy the chair and drive it down to Atlanta for a birthday present. This plan has already been made before the movie starts. We begin *in medias res*, as Josh and his girlfriend Emily are discussing the trip. She wants to come; he doesn't really want her to. Things escalate, they argue, and she leaves. The next morning, he turns up outside her apartment, tells her he loves her and that he does want her to come. They hit the road, and the story is now about their relationship.

Of course, you can argue that their argument is the inciting incident—it is the dramatic incident that leads to Emily being included in the road trip, after all. But the movie clearly refers that argument back to the original plan, that we pick up on through their conversation. It's like we come into the movie watching the second beat. We have already had the inciting incident and now we are into the debate. Do we need to have things spelled out for us? No.

Multi-plot movies usually have single inciting incidents that resonate across all the plots (or multiple, if thematically connected incidents initiate each strand). For example, *Love Actually* opens with shots of people greeting each other in the arrivals hall at Heathrow Airport. We hear David in voice-over talking about how "love is everywhere," thus establishing the theme of the movie. Then we work our way around the rest of the characters and discover they are all dealing with love in one way or another. Their plot threads are free to develop independently, as we have already been instructed how to read the movie.

DO YOU REALLY HAVE 10 MINUTES TO HOOK 'EM?

The further your writing diverges from the Hollywood norm, the less you need to pay attention to this issue. The same applies if you are working in television, where more and more shows are allowed to start "slow." On the other hand, if you need big budget financing for a Hollywood genre movie, you probably have around ten pages to grab the reader's attention.

Studio realities also answer why we need to "hook 'em" in the first place: If you don't make the agent or producer want to read past page 10 of your screenplay, then they probably won't. If you are an A-list writer and have a personal relationship with your agent, they might read on. But if you are submitting a spec script for coverage, then you need to get a reader engaged early if you want that all-important grade of "consider" on the report.

Pacing and Today's Media

The question of pacing is another example of the impact of media convergence on creative screen storytelling. On the one hand, genre movie storytelling has accelerated since the 1970s. It used to be the case that genre movies could use relatively slow-burning first acts to build conflict and context together.

Now, common practice is to open with a bang—sometimes literally—and drive on from there. If you compare *Poltergeist* (1982) with its 2015 remake, this could not be clearer. In the original, the first act is slow, as we get to know and care about the family who will be haunted.

In contrast, the 2015 remake has weird stuff happening in the house from the first night.

There are exceptions. *Arrival* (2016) frontloads its first act with a major catalytic event: the alien spaceships appear. But then things move relatively slowly as the communication research project gets underway. Of course, *Arrival* considers itself a serious science-fiction film, not a big-budget exploitation movie. As a rule, however, contemporary Hollywood genre storytelling starts fast and accelerates.

Worthy, character-led dramas and high-profile, Oscar-bait productions are somewhat less frenetic. Even so, many of these are also briskly paced. *Little Women* (2019), adapted and directed by Greta Gerwig, was one of my favorite films of the last few years, and it was driven on by snappy scene work and the dynamism of its performances. That pacing feels organic because the intelligence of the characters encourages us to want to experience storytelling at the pace of their perspicacity.

WHAT IS A PLOT ARC?

A plot arc, similar to a story arc, is a continuing narrative strand that unfolds through your movie. In episodic television, it indicates that a particular story issue—a relationship, a quest, etc.—will play out over multiple episodes or even seasons. In the TV show *Battlestar Galactica* (2004–2009), the primary arc is about the human fleet seeking Earth. In movies, a plot or story arc can refer to the main story or to a subplot. Either way, the arc is established, plays out, and is resolved at or near the end.

When the term is related to a character, it usually refers to the narrative of change or development that they go through during the course of the movie. The audience mentally marks that change when the character does something revealing. At the end of the movie, the character's arc is resolved in relationship to their theme. Along the way, we most commonly mark its development through the character's changing relationships with other characters.

To get you started in your thinking, we are going to begin by focusing on two clear and simple ways of conceiving your story:

1. From plot to character.

2. From character to plot.

From Plot to Character

Plot trumps character in a wide range of movies, from a genre classic like *Mad Max 2: The Road Warrior* (1981) to the journalism drama *Spotlight* (2015). Remember that just because a movie is plot-led doesn't mean it should have one-note or poorly written characters. Similarly, a plot-driven film isn't somehow intrinsically lesser than a character-led movie.

Remember *San Andreas* (2015)? Even if we are fans of the talented cast, *San Andreas* is a plot-driven disaster movie. I'm willing to bet that project started from plot and worked its way to character. Nonetheless, if we are telling an effects-heavy earthquake fable, we need to know who the survivors are and how we can make them interesting enough to be invested in their survival. We still need that simple human story—it is the emotional glue that binds the movie together.

From Character to Plot

When we think about story development from character to plot, we begin with a fascinating character and then build a plot for them to explore their dramatic potential. The most obvious example would be a biopic, but a character-led film can be any type of movie in which the personalities of the protagonists and antagonists and their conflicts drive those stories. Examples range from the slow-paced, human-boy-befriends-child-vampire film *Let the Right One In/Låt den rätte komma in* (2008) to the first John Rambo movie, *First Blood* (1982), in which the persecuted Vietnam vet spends a good part of the movie injuring law enforcement officers with his improvised booby traps.

How Do I Know If It's a Good Plot?

There's a big difference between a cool image, or a cool sequence, and a cool story. You can imagine an earthquake movie with skyscrapers falling and cars driving into giant crevices in the ground, but what will sustain our interest? The answer is that great characters sustain our interest. Ask yourself: Who can be at the heart of this idea?

Let's work that earthquake disaster movie concept a little harder. *San Andreas* gave the lead to a helicopter rescue pilot, which was smart because he has the skills to help and the transport to fly over the destruction to get to where he's going. But what if we have no helicopters? If you're the screenwriter, then it's your job to think about other viable ways to tell a California earthquake story. You can populate the concept with characters to test it.

Say that in our *San Andreas* movie, we are trapped in an underground train. You have the potential for an ensemble movie with all the survivors. There would be people of different races, genders, ages, and economic backgrounds, because everyone wants to beat the traffic. But was the train going east or west—toward San Francisco or the East Bay? And what time of day is it when your story begins? That might have an impact on who had boarded the train. Is your movie a hybrid genre? Are there criminals on the train? A monster? A serial killer? Or is this a straightforward escape-and-survival story, with a clock as the railway starts to collapse? Any of these options can work, but each potentially has a different cast of characters and different story priorities.

Assuming it's a survival story, maybe your protagonist can be a young girl who has the brains, the guts, and the small body to get through the tight spaces in the crushed train car and find help for herself and the injured adults she leaves behind. Maybe you scale the threats down to her size and experience. A big rat becomes very scary if you are nine years old, to say nothing of a whole pack. Her fellow passengers ask her to try and get out because none of them can fit. Her mother is injured, she is unconscious and can't help; so our young heroine is on her own.

Or maybe she's a teenage runaway. Maybe her family lost their home through gentrification and are living out of their car. There's no way this girl will trust the techies who are being loud and obnoxious on the train.

The next thing you can ask yourself: How do I make a hackneyed old plot device new and interesting? Class war on the trapped train car? This question brings us to strong characters. And, from there, a twist. Eventually, questions around plot, subplot, and character will bring you home to theme. Your theme gives everyone and everything in your story focus, and that's what you need to tie up your creative threads.

PLOTS AND SUBPLOTS

For clarity and ease of communication, in Hollywood screenwriting, key plot or story strands have identifying letters. The most important two are the A story and the B story (even though there will likely be more than two strands in your script). Both these terms have specific meanings and they are also focused around your story's theme, as we shall see.

A Stories

In Hollywood, the A story is always the lead plot strand. Specifically, A stories deal with what the protagonist wants in the plot. It is about surface motivation and practical achievements: "I need to do X."

In a romantic comedy, for example, the A story is the central romantic relationship: Girl meets girl, boy meets boy, person meets person, and in any event those crazy kids try to make it work. In the A story, a problem is revealed, which the protagonist has to try and resolve: Girl meets girl, but Girl 2 is a nun. Or married. Or an alien. Boy meets boy, but Boy 2 is way out of his league. Or a serial killer. Or hiding a secret. If it was easy, it wouldn't be a story. The A story relates to emotions—our girl protagonist *really* likes that other girl—but it focuses on the practical challenges of the relationship.

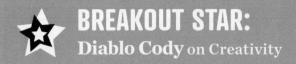

BREAKOUT STAR:
Diablo Cody on Creativity

In this chapter we are thinking about where ideas come from and how to discipline them. In a 2011 interview with Collider, Diablo Cody, the screenwriter who won an Oscar for *Juno* (2007), discusses the slanted yet personal origins of many of her ideas:

"The things that I write are autobiographical in a surreal sense, like when you have a dream and you go to the doctor's office, but then you turn around and it's actually your childhood home and the doctor has turned into Ryan Reynolds. You know what I mean? You have these dreams that are about an essential truth in your life, but they're also just totally garbled and creative and strange. The stuff I write isn't strictly autobiographical, but it's personal, if that makes any sense. It draws all these little incidents and people out of my life and then contorts them."

In Hollywood movies, the problem in the plot parallels a problem in the story. There is an internal conflict, challenge, or lack that your protagonist has to overcome to be able to resolve the problem in the A story plotline. This prompts soul-searching or testing and leads to character change. As we have already noted, we can't *see* internal conflict on the screen, so it has to be worked through externally, through relationships with other characters. That's where we get to the B story.

B Stories

We call the key character relationship through which we get privileged access to our protagonist's thoughts and feelings the B story.

The B story relationship can be a friendship, a family relationship, or a mentoring relationship. Most commonly, however, the B story is a romantic subplot—only not the lead romance in a romantic comedy, as we just established. Why do B stories exist? Well, who do *you* confide in? I'm guessing your answer is probably a friend, a family member, an advisor, or a lover. It's the people with whom you are the most open and vulnerable, the people whom you trust the most.

The B story comes into play most strongly in the second act of a screenplay—the act that is all about character change. Our protagonist checks in with the B story character regularly, and that's how we know what they are feeling, and how they are making progress toward resolving their inner conflict. Typically, the B story character actively helps them along, in any number of ways.

The B story resolves at the end of act two, when the B story character helps the protagonist formulate the plan they will follow in act three to resolve the A story. (It's okay if you need to map this out.) Remember that the B story character may turn up in all three acts, but their role in the B story relationship is focused around act two.

The Rest of the Alphabet

Every other plotline and relationship in your movie can be given a letter to identify it, but there is nothing special about these. Only A and B (and maybe C; see below) mean something specific. Remember, however, that well-written subplots are very important because they inform, support, and help to pay off your main story. They enrich your script and give us context and depth that your A story is too busy to deliver.

Some writers use the term "C story" to refer to the protagonist's character arc. In this version, if the A story is the plot and the B story is an emotional relationship, then the C story is where we see the protagonist change and develop. This is not a universal model, however, and many writers just work with A and B, whereas C becomes just another subplot strand.

PLOT STRANDS IN TV

In TV writing, the letters have a somewhat different meaning. The A story will be the primary plot of the episode, getting the most scenes and screen time. The B story is usually either a parallel plot for supporting characters, or the emotional story strand for the leads that runs alongside the A story. It gets the second-most screen time.

The other letters of the alphabet are assigned to what are sometimes called "runners"—ongoing plot threads that link this episode to the rest of the season and pay off entirely in the future or as a drip feed across episodes. In television comedies, the C story may also refer to running gags.

Different shows may use the strands for different purposes, although the basic model holds. A show could use the A story for drama, and the B story for comic relief, for example. Typically, no matter the choices here, the A and B stories will interact.

THE ROLE OF THEME

In a reductive sense, almost all movies are led by their theme. Theme drives character, story, and plot. Without a consistent theme, your story will meander in unhelpful and confusing ways and will end up being unsatisfying to an audience. We are not always aware of a story's theme as we are watching, especially when the theme is implicit and isn't foregrounded as a major structural marker, but it is always there.

Of course, there are also movies that make a big issue out of their theme. *Invictus* (2009), the movie about South Africa winning the Rugby World Cup, is clearly led by its linked themes of forgiveness and reconciliation. *Braveheart* (1995) is about many things, including revenge, bad hair, and blue face paint, but you may recall that it is also about "Freedom!" We know this because Mel Gibson takes the trouble to remind us (in a very loud voice).

Theme drives your story, which will shape your screenplay. Regardless of the structural road your movie follows, the theme will inform the film's goals. Here are some vital things to consider as you begin your story development:

- What does your protagonist want?
- What are they struggling with and against?
- Is your theme love, betrayal, loyalty, growing up, friendship, revenge, survival?

All of these themes, and many more, are great because they push your characters to make active choices that drive them to action and that move your story forward. Remember that just because the plot of your movie is about a love affair doesn't mean its theme is love. It can just as easily be about courage, freedom, oppression, or grief. We'll do an exercise on the storytelling power of themes later in this chapter.

Themes also give characters attitudes. If your theme is love, then ask yourself, what does my protagonist think about love at the start and at the end? How has the journey of the story changed them in this regard, if at all? When your protagonist has an attitude about love, then you can begin to populate your story with other attitudes that create tension and conflict. In other words, attitudes—in relationship to your theme—drive your story.

If your protagonist is naïve and believes in love at first sight while their best friend is more cynical, well, that gives you some interesting potential for character interaction right off the bat. You can riff from there: What is their love interest's attitude? How about the love interest's best friend? There's a whole screenplay's worth of drama just in the interactions of those four characters and their attitudes toward love. This can lead to bigger theme-related questions or dilemmas: Are your lovers their own worst enemies? Is their story really about the love between friends? In the writing process, it's helpful to explicitly sketch out your theme for yourself, and then let theme inform the direction of your writing. You don't want to write a screenplay and go back to look for the theme later.

The Sweet Spot

Once you've landed on your theme, it won't change. Hear this again: Your theme never changes, but attitudes to it will.

Your story may be about many ideas or events, but it only has one articulating theme. That theme keeps you honest and organized all the way until the end of your script. If your theme changes, you are writing a different story. When this happens, it's confusing and unsatisfying for your audience. Similarly, a theme that is too general or passive won't be much help. You have to ask: "How do I drive this theme?" When you know the answer to that question, you might have a workable theme.

There are many stories you can tell about a character, but this one is about how they fell in love—or how they dealt with betrayal, growing up, etc. Similarly, your protagonist might start the story as naïve and grow into cynicism as they experience the reality of a relationship, or they might start your story swearing off relationships only to find that true love melts their cold heart. Once you understand your characters' goals and your movie's theme, the hard part is getting the reader to take a journey that is both logical and enjoyable from premise to conclusion.

Common Themes

Everything we have discussed so far in your story development comes together in your theme. All we need to do to integrate our inciting incident, our A story, our B story, and our other subplots is to articulate a theme. Then every part of your story will move in the same direction, even if your characters are cussed contrarians. The reason we discuss them in this order is that to view the theme without a catalyst or plot threads, there is nothing to tie its meaning together.

Rather than discussing theme in the abstract, let's run some common movie themes though a hypothetical story and do the work. I have come up with a basic science fiction concept as our test bed for different themes, but also remember that each of these examples is only one way that the theme could drive your story.

Keep in mind that while a movie story has one dominant theme, a theme that keeps your storytelling honest, it may not be the only theme in your story. Can a movie be about coming of age and love? Yes, but only one of those themes *drives* the story. Similarly, it is likely that many of these themes will overlap.

Here's our situation: little Jimmy O'Toole is a middle-school-aged kid in suburban Philadelphia. His mom is deceased and his dad is a struggling single parent. Jimmy acts out. Then, one night, he arrives home after playing on bikes with his friends to find his dad being taken on board a spaceship in the backyard. Jimmy stows away on the alien ship, determined to rescue his dad, only to find that this is no alien abduction. His father is in a romantic relationship with the captain of the spaceship and is leaving Earth—at least temporarily—for interstellar adventures, romantic and otherwise. Now let's run that very simple idea through different themes; they each shift our perspective a little and even offer ideas for the plot.

COMING OF AGE

Little Jimmy is growing up, but that brings challenges of all sorts. His job will be to accept that his father is his own person and deserves to be happy. He will also grow as a person in coming to terms with his dad's relationship, such that he might be ready for one of his own.

LOVE

Jimmy's dad and Captain Shiny (the dashing space captain, keep up) are truly in love. They were going to tell him eventually, but they were wrapped up in the romance. It takes a while for Jimmy to understand. It takes a bit longer for him to forgive his dad. But the captain's cute niece is also on the ship. Maybe she can teach Jimmy a thing or two about space dating, so there's an upside.

SACRIFICE

Jimmy has made a terrible mistake. He has been a selfish little brat. He comes to understand the sacrifices his father has made for him and determines that he owes him a major sacrifice of his own. He will risk everything for him to be happy. His dad is a widower, but did his mother sacrifice herself for them in some way?

PERSEVERANCE

Jimmy is a real brat, but he's a tough little brat. When he realizes how he's let his father down, he will stop at nothing to make amends. The movie will test him to the utmost. Jimmy's change happens early in the story but once he has made it—good luck getting in his way.

FAMILY

This is a catch-all and encompasses much of the rest of the story. The key here is that Jimmy doesn't value family at the start of the movie—his mom is dead, families fall apart, only suckers invest emotionally in their family. But maybe there can be a new family for the O'Tooles in the future—and isn't the mismatched alien crew of the spaceship a kind of family? Jimmy changes his view of what a family can and should be. He learns the value of family as the story progresses.

FRIENDSHIP

Captain Shiny must be a villain, because she wants to take Jimmy's dad away and make him betray the memory of his mom. Actually, she's not a bad person, and when Jimmy finally comes to accept that, oh the adventures they'll have together. Part of that theme is Jimmy coming to view his father as a person. Here's a heretic thought: Maybe your dad can be your friend as well.

REVENGE

Jimmy learns that his family is not from Earth. They are refugees from an evil space villain who killed Jimmy's mom. Now Jimmy is on a quest for vengeance, unless his dad can help him see another way.

JUSTICE

As above, but now revenge is moderated into bringing the villain to account.

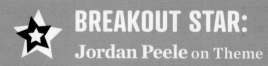

BREAKOUT STAR:
Jordan Peele on Theme

Below, Jordan Peele, the writer/director of *Us* (2019) and *Get Out* (2017), for which he won a screenwriting Academy Award, offers insights into the thematic implications of his movie for black horror audiences in particular. Theme speaks to character, but it also attempts to evoke a particular kind of identification, as he explained to Slash Film:

"As far as the visual motifs of the film, one of the themes is neglect. It is that which we sort of stuff to the back of our minds. One of the satirical but, I think, powerful notes that the movie hits is this idea of being in a dark room where there is a reality happening on a screen in front of us, and you can yell and you can scream and you can shout, but you're not going to change what happens in that world on that screen. That to me is a metaphor for, among other things, the lack of representation of black people and a black perspective in a horror film, a genre that black people are very loyal to. Of course, you know the stereotype of going to a black theater and watching and hearing the black audience yelling, 'Get out. Turn around. Bitch, call the cops.' That to me, in essence, is a form of the sunken place, which is in the movie. It is a de-marginalization, so that's just one, but there's a lot of layers going on."

CLIMAXING—AND OTHER ALTERNATIVES

In the three-act paradigm, a movie's climax resolves the theme. Girl keeps girl. Boy keeps boy. Good triumphs. Evil is defeated. We live happily ever after—unless it's a tearjerker, and then we still have the nobility of sacrifice or heroic endurance to draw from. At least, that's how it works in a mainstream movie. When everything ends happily, that's an "up ending." If it all ends tragically, that's a "down ending." It's nothing like real life, but everything you need for a Hollywood redemptive ending.

In order to check if your climax is working properly for goal-driven protagonists, answer these questions:

1. Does my antagonist effectively oppose the theme of the movie, and is it clear that their defeat also represents the resolution of that theme?

2. In defeating my antagonist and resolving the theme, does my protagonist do something that they could not have pulled off in act one? In other words, did they develop and change?

3. Does the climax of my story resolve both the plot and the story of the film?

At the end of *Little Women*, Jo March makes a deal to publish her book. She shows her cleverness and determination by negotiating good royalties and keeping copyright, ensuring ongoing income from her writing labor. She also inherits her aunt's house and opens it as a school, thus providing gainful employment for her sisters.

This ending clearly resolves the theme of independence that the March sisters, and especially Jo, have been struggling with throughout the story. In particular, it resolves the primary question that writer/director Greta Gerwig poses through her characters: What are the economic conditions for women who truly want to be independent? Jo gains her economic freedom, but to achieve it she has to change the ending of her own book. It is a sacrifice that she deems worth making, and one that brings a healthy dose of realism to the up ending.

This ending also resolves the challenge of the antagonistic force in the movie, which I would describe as economic dependence. It threatens the March family in many ways and is embodied in a range of characters. With Jo's success, they are free of it at last.

MOVING AWAY FROM MAINSTREAM ENDINGS

The farther we get from the mainstream, the more ambivalent, contingent, contradictory, or "realistic" a story's resolution may be. Remember that the climax of a movie may embody different outcomes in the story and the plot. The world may be saved, for example, but our protagonist may have suffered to achieve it.

For an inventive ambivalent ending, look to Rian Johnson's terrific hard-boiled high school detective movie, *Brick* (2005). In the film, an outsider high school kid named Brendan discovers the body of his ex-girlfriend and sets out to find the killer. He succeeds. By the end, he brings justice, of a kind, both to the boy who killed her and the girl (the antagonist and femme fatale) who manipulated him into doing it. But the investigation has cost Brendan a lot. He has internal injuries from repeated beatings, and he has uncovered very ugly truths about the people closest to him.

In the end, we can say that Brendan has succeeded in the plot—there is an up ending that reveals justice. But there is also a down ending in the story due to what it cost. Physically and psychologically, Brendan is kind of broken, and he will certainly never be the same again. The ending is ambivalent, and our emotional response likely also conflicted. In this way, *Brick*'s ending is more realistic, under a certain definition of realism, than many Hollywood endings.

In the Writers' Room:
INCITING INCIDENT EXERCISE

For this exercise, we are going to ask the important question: What kind of inciting incident works best for your theme?

Remember little Jimmy and his fraught relationship with his dad? Well, let's think through a couple of ways that story could open. There are many options, of course, and I'm going to offer notes toward one version for each of our go-to iterations of the inciting incident.

THE CHARACTER-DRIVEN MODEL:

We open on little Jimmy out playing with his buddies on bikes. (I know, it's the law, right?) Meanwhile, Jimmy's dad is cleaning the house. We follow him, revealing evidence that he's a widower (photographs, etc.).

Cut back: Jimmy rides aggressively, doing tricks and taking risks. These are dynamic action scenes. Opening with a bang.

Quick scene. Dad still cleaning. Jimmy's room is a mess. Evidence of Jimmy's anger: His taste in music, his scary art . . .

The kids get thirsty and arrive at Jimmy's house to raid the fridge. Jimmy's dad tries to be friendly, but the kids ignore him. He asks them: "Please don't leave a m . . ."—they leave a mess. Dad is alone again, depressed amid the debris. Night falls. Lights come on in the neighborhood as Jimmy rides home. Jimmy and Dad eat dinner in silence. Jimmy goes to bed. Listens to punk rock on his headphones. Falls asleep listening. Dad watches TV. He grabs

CONTINUED ▶

the remote and presses buttons. Only, that doesn't look like any remote control we've ever seen. Jimmy wakes to lights and noise outside. He goes to the window and there's a spaceship in his yard.

THE (AMBIVALENT) COINCIDENCE MODEL:

We open on Jimmy out playing with his buddies on bikes. (It's still the law.) Jimmy rides aggressively, doing tricks and taking risks. Dynamic action scene. Jimmy's friends worry at his risk-taking. It is getting dark. One by one they take off for home until it's just Jimmy and his best friend, Seth. Seth says, "I gotta go. My parents will be worried." Jimmy: "Pfft, who cares?" Jimmy stays out in the darkening streets doing tricks until he can't see. He falls and scrapes his knee. No tears, he's a tough little kid, but he heads home to see noise and lights. There's a spaceship in his yard. Jimmy pedals furiously, when he's closer he sees his dad silhouetted in the hatchway. He sees Jimmy, points. Jimmy: "Dad!"

See the difference? Of course, you can like my openings or hate them, but they play very differently because of how much we know about the father. In the first version, we understand Jimmy's dad's frustration and it will make sense when we understand later that he's leaving—even if it's just for his regular date night with Captain Shiny. We also figure out pretty quickly that he was calling her on the "remote." In the second version, we get that Jimmy has some issues, but we know nothing about his dad. The "abduction" plays like a coincidence and all the tasty reveals are saved for later.

In our example, is it more fun to sympathize with Dad and wait for Jimmy to get a clue or to identify with

Jimmy and enjoy the shocks of the reveals? There is no simple and universal correct answer to this, but the way your story will play on your audience will be significantly different depending on your choice here. This is a part of narration—the impact your storytelling choices have on your audience's engagement with your story.

For this exercise, simply try both versions of inciting incident with your own story. Beat out the opening for both and see which you prefer.

CREATE SOMEONE TO ROOT FOR

Is "hero" just another word for "protagonist"? Well, the answer is yes and no. In general, we associate the word "hero" with bravery. And although bravery comes in many forms, not all protagonists are truly brave.

Many protagonists start out a long way from heroism. As we now know, in conventional three-act models of movie storytelling the midpoint includes a second and profound commitment to action on behalf of our protagonist. This is precisely the point that often turns mere protagonists into heroes. By this time, the protagonist has already learned or experienced enough to understand the true consequences of their decision. Deciding to move forward toward their goal, despite knowing how bad things are likely to get, is the courageous act that makes them a hero.

Of course, not all stories treat bravery or heroism in the same way. What they share is a commitment to goals. Let's have a look.

GOAL-DRIVEN CHARACTERS

We may think of this as adherence to a theme, as wants, or as needs, but whatever words we use to describe these characters, they come under the tried and true category of goal-driven heroes in goal-led stories.

The three-act paradigm is designed to tell goal-led stories. In fact, the structure assumes you are developing your characters for exactly that purpose. Goal-driven characters are, almost by definition, dynamic and inclined to push forward in search of that end, no matter how unlikely it might seem that they can achieve it. Consequently, one of the most enjoyable—if also unrealistic—aspects of most Hollywood stories is the ability of their goal-driven heroes to change from unworthy or incapable to worthy and capable within the space of three acts.

Not all stories work their characters in exactly this way. By the end of the first act, Conan is already stronger than we can imagine and the rest of the movie tests his strength and resilience. Likewise, the Elizabeth of the 2005 adaptation (if not Jane Austen's original) doesn't transform from loser to winner in this narrow sense; rather, she learns to overcome her negative views (her prejudice) about Darcy when he proves himself worthy of her love. It is still character change, however, and a significant one in the terms of her story.

Character Change

We will discuss other models of movie character in the next section but, for now, one requirement of writing good goal-driven characters is to establish what constitutes appropriate change in your story. How, and how much, do your heroes need to develop morally, physically, or otherwise in order to achieve their goals? What is their range of change?

Every story establishes a different scale by which we judge character development, and we will return to this in another form when we discuss changing archetypes in the next chapter. For now, this is a simple principle to help you position goal-driven heroes in your stories: The range within which we measure character change is established by their opening condition and capped by their story goal.

SAGE SPOTLIGHT:
Callie Khouri on
Writing Characters

Callie Khouri, the screenwriter who won an Oscar for *Thelma and Louise* (1991), talked to the late, great screenwriting teacher Syd Field about her process. The sense that she describes of being open to your characters and waiting for them to speak to you is something many writers share.

"Once I have thought out the action of the story, and have a handle on the characters, I'll go out in the backyard in the morning, and just sit there and try to open myself up and let the characters come to me; let them talk to me. So much of writing is about getting quiet enough so you can hear your characters talking. Sometimes I feel they choose you because they know you're listening. You just have to shut up and listen. My greatest challenge was not to impose myself on them and just let them say what they've got to say. If I'm in turmoil about what a character is doing, I have to be careful not to let my own turmoil destroy what's happening. It's very much a miscommunication between me and them. The same way it would be with a real person."

Goal-driven protagonists are also common in independent features. We just have to adjust our vision to see their "small" changes at the magnification they deserve. For example, your shy protagonist who can't talk to girls ends up having a proper conversation with one. They aren't dating—maybe they aren't even friends (yet)—but he got through it without making an ass of himself. He's learned to do it. He's earned it. That's big progress in the terms of *his* story. He may not have killed a gang of Russian mobsters along the way like John Wick, but we can still see him as heroic.

THE ANTIHERO OR ALTERNATIVE PROTAGONIST

"Antihero" is a rather old-fashioned term for a flawed or unconventional protagonist whose moral character and actions are less than admirable, more equivocal, or even in some ways actively evil. We may still admire them because, for all their flaws, they do the right thing, even if they do it for the "wrong" reasons.

Alternatively, we may not admire them, but secretly wish we were more like them because they are cool, or powerful, or just because they don't give a damn what the world thinks of them. Iconic movie antiheroes—like Patrick Bateman in *American Psycho* (2000), "Joe," aka the Man With No Name from *A Fistful of Dollars/Per un pugno di dollari* (1964), Lisbeth Salander in *The Girl with the Dragon Tattoo/Män som hatar kvinnor* (2009), and Harley Quinn from *Birds of Prey: And the Fantabulous Emancipation of One Harley Quinn* (2020)—are exciting precisely because they break rules and often act independent of conventional morality.

But antiheroes are not the only alternatives to classic goal-driven Hollywood protagonists. There are two important ways we can set up these alternatives. The first is to go back to the Greeks and think of a character not as a person as much as a dramatic function. The second is to look at the work of independent, avant-garde, and countercultural screenwriters and filmmakers who tell stories in which characters have very different motivations and purposes than they do in your typical Hollywood tentpole movie.

Let's start with the Greeks. When Aristotle discusses "character" in *Poetics*, he subordinates it in importance to plot. The action of a tragedy is the most important aspect of drama; character comes in second. Moreover, he uses words to describe character that are not, strictly speaking, evoking a person at all. A full discussion of Aristotle's ideas is beyond the scope of this book, but let's go over a couple of important principles to give you a different perspective on what characters are and how they work.

The Shifting Protagonist

In his book *Me and You and Memento and Fargo*, J. J. Murphy uses the example of Jerry Lundegaard and Marge Gunderson in the Coen brothers' *Fargo* (1996) to discuss the challenge of shifting protagonists. Fargo is a multiple-plot movie, a relatively common storytelling strategy in 1990s indie filmmaking. In this movie, we move back and forth between Jerry's ransom scheme and Marge's attempt to investigate murders as a law enforcement officer. Some film buffs argue *Fargo* is an ensemble movie, but Murphy correctly notes the amount of time we spend with Jerry and Marge and the weight the story gives to their separate actions. The movie works precisely because they are both protagonists of their own plot—the role of protagonist, in other words, shifts from one to the other. Shifting protagonists are very rare.

Character, According to Aristotle

When Aristotle speaks of character, he uses the Greek word *ethos*. Ethos is broadly translated as moral character, and it sits alongside *dianoia*, or the process of logical thought. Aristotle uses the term ethos in his book *Poetics* to signify the key motivator for change in drama. What's important is how ethos prompts a character to act.

Praxis is another Greek word that refers to the deeds or actions a person does. Remember that for Aristotle, action is more important than character, therefore praxis is more important than ethos. Some important screenwriters and teachers follow this principle. The screenwriting teacher Robert McKee famously wrote in *Story* that "character is action."

The playwright and screenwriter David Mamet put it even more forcefully in his book *On Directing Film* when he said there was no such thing as character: "It doesn't exist. The character is just habitual action."

This is a provocative and important idea, especially when we remember that cinema is a visual medium. We don't have access to internal dialogue, so we judge a character by what they say and, more importantly, by what they do. Thinking of character as praxis is not necessarily an alternative to the idea of the goal-driven protagonist, but rather it underpins any kind of movie character because of the nature of the medium.

Praxis occurs at different levels of drama. It can involve big acts that drive a story forward—moments of violence are a common form of praxis in Hollywood movies. But praxis is also bound up in all the tiny tells of non-verbal communication that reveal character in subtle but important ways. Sometimes this is found in performance, but it can be important work for a screenwriter as well.

An example of a character who communicates to the audience mostly through non-verbal means would be Chance the gardener, played by Peter Sellers in *Being There* (1979). A simple and quiet man, when he speaks he is often misunderstood by people who have their own, usually political motivations for doing so. Another example, from a very different kind of movie, would be the mute gunfighter, Silence, in Sergio Corbucci's spaghetti western *The Great Silence/Il grande silenzio* (1968).

In the end, all characters are defined by praxis, even the loquacious ones. After all, praxis also has a verbal component. We learn a great deal about characters not only from what they say, but how they say it. (We'll learn even more about this when we deal with dialogue in rule 10.)

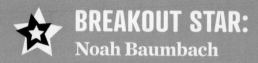

BREAKOUT STAR:
Noah Baumbach

Noah Baumbach, writer and director of *The Squid and the Whale* (2005), *Greenberg* (2010), and *Marriage Story* (2019), is known for chronicling the lives of characters who are unconventional for movies but do seem more like real people. Baumbach makes this point eloquently in an interview with Anthony Kaufman for IndieWire:

"I really feel these characters are a lot like people in the world. They're only 'difficult' compared to conventional movie characters. I don't think they're difficult compared to real human beings. I'm surprised how people react so strongly. Their argument is, 'Who is like this?' But they don't realize they're using other movies as comparison rather than using their own parents or themselves."

BACKSTORY (OR, WHAT ALL PROTAGONISTS HAVE IN COMMON)

The term "backstory" refers to a character's past. Backstory is important because every character you write had a life before at least some of the events of your story began. Screenwriters focus on backstories because a character's life experience informs and motivates their actions in the present moment of every scene they're in.

I'm writing this section on a pleasant February morning in Santa Rosa, California. I'm sitting in my office at home and listening to the dog scratching on the door because he wants a walk (he can wait for a bit). My personal writing style emerges from a series of conscious decisions—I'm trying to come off as helpful, informed, and yet chatty and accessible. How's it working? In so doing, I am drawing on specific areas of my knowledge, my experience, and my personality. I am making conscious connections with memories and skills that are part of my sense of who I am, what I've done, the movies I've watched, written, consulted on, and, in a general sense, what I know. For example, I just gave myself the choice between writing that the dog can "chill for now" or "wait for a bit." (As a transplanted Englishman I went for what felt like the more UK English option.) Again, that was a conscious choice.

But my writing is also informed in ways that are less immediately obvious to me, but that might be revealing to you. Things like the vocabulary I use, my turn of phrase, my (sometimes questionable) syntax and so forth probably reveal clues about my education, cultural background, gender, class, and no doubt many other "tells" of which I am not as keenly aware.

It's the same with characters in a story. A character will reflect their past as they act in the present. That reflection is a combination of big things, like the resentment they feel toward the police because of how they were frequently stopped and frisked, and small things, like the fact they were a fan of Taylor Swift at the age of 12 and nobody in their family understood why. Do both of these things matter equally for your story? Not necessarily. But they might both play a role.

In the abstract, we might assume resentment toward the police is a more important thing to know than being a ridiculed childhood fan of a pop star, but our story could have nothing to do with the police and everything to do with family relationships where nobody lets our protagonist forget his childhood obsessions. In our story, our friend is never taken seriously by his family because he was something of a cultural misfit and, now that he's approaching adulthood and wants to assert himself into family decision-making, that's his struggle.

The example raises the two key questions about backstory:

- What do you need to know to write a good character?
- What does the audience need to know about them to engage with your story?

These questions often have different answers, and many ways to get to the bottom of each one. For now, this rule should guide you: Backstory is important when it impacts how your character will interact with the theme of the story.

In the Writers' Room:
CHARACTER BACKSTORY EXERCISE

Backstory is tricky. If your thinking isn't disciplined, you can get lost in the details. This exercise is aimed at making sure that the backstory you create for a character serves your story and does justice to your theme.

First, come up with a protagonist for a story you are working on, or one you can imagine for this exercise. If your story has multiple or shared protagonists, pick one. (You can always do it again with the others later.)

Answer these two preparatory questions first:

1. What is your story's theme?
2. What does your protagonist have to do in the story to advance and resolve that theme?

Next, answer these questions about backstory, given your answers to the two questions above:

1. How does your protagonist's family background impact their views?
2. How does their life experience prepare them to be who they need to be in the story?

In answering the second question, consider the following: their profession, their past romantic or friend relationships (including with other characters in the movie), their education, their experience of success or failure, their traumas, their personal, cultural, and moral values. Give yourself permission to discount

CONTINUED ►

anything that doesn't let you make a direct and powerful connection with the theme of the story.

Finally, now that you know something about your protagonist and how their past is a prologue, work in a less detailed backstory for all the other major characters who have influenced or who will change the trajectory of the protagonist's life on screen.

INVESTIGATE ARCHETYPES

So far, we have discussed goal-driven characters—
the most common type of Hollywood movie
character—and we have broached the idea that characters serve your story's theme.

In this rule, we are still focused on characters, but
now we are going to consider another way of popu-
lating your screenplay by thinking of characters in
terms of the roles they play in your story. This brings
us to archetypes.

PROCEED, BUT WITH CAUTION

Whether or not you decide to incorporate archetypes in your writing, there is value in examining the technique. Some of the most powerful and popular characters in literature and film—Atticus Finch in *To Kill a Mockingbird* (1962), Luke Skywalker in *Star Wars*, Ripley in *Alien*—embody archetypes. Knowing how they work can structure your writing process and help generate ideas, even if you decide approaching characters through archetypes is not for you.

The goal is to learn from the technique, not to become beholden to it. It's good to be skeptical of archetypes, though, because it is easy to write stereotypical characters by using them. At the end of this chapter, you can find an exercise to keep you on track, but it's something to be aware of so that you can catch yourself.

With that said, let's see how some of the best screenwriting teachers use archetypes. We are going to look at two influential variants on the model—one from John Truby, author of *The Anatomy of Story*, and the other from Christopher Vogler, author of *The Writer's Journey*. There is a lot of overlap between them, but also some important distinctions. Both books are smart and useful, and Vogler's works especially well if you are developing mythic, fantasy, or science fiction stories.

WHAT ARE ARCHETYPES?

I'm certainly not an expert on Carl Jung's psychoanalytic theory, the basis for archetypes, but essentially, he proposed that an archetype is a kind of inherited psychological pattern within an individual. It is linked to the idea of a "collective unconscious": unconscious structures that are supposedly shared by all human beings. Because of this collective unconscious, the theory goes, at birth our individual consciousness is not a clean slate, and our identities as individuals are inflected by the common species material our psyches inherit.

Archetypes are powerful, shared, and innate symbols embedded in our collective unconscious. They are universal symbols, recognized in some deep way by us all.

We don't have to buy into Jung's theories to use archetypes as a writing tool. For many screenwriters, the concept has been useful because archetypes focus on the key role or function that a person plays in the world of a screenplay. As a first step in inventing a character, giving them an active purpose is a useful thing. A Trickster uses her wits to get what she wants, for example. She may have the gift of gab and be persuasive; she may be a lying con artist (or both). Either way, you have a big clue as to how she operates—and what motivates her to do so.

The idea is that archetypes can be fairly universal. For example, the Warrior archetype still holds whether your character is a samurai, an Amazonian, or a US marine. Similarly, the Mentor archetype includes Gandalf from *The Lord of the Rings* trilogy (2001–2003), Jiminy Cricket in *Pinocchio* (1940), and Jimmy Dugan in *A League of Their Own* (1992), who famously reminded us that: "There's no crying in baseball." As you can tell from the breadth of those examples, archetypes should encourage your creativity when you are building characters within them, not restrict it. Remember: Not all Mentors are like Yoda, and not all Tricksters are like Loki.

Archetypes in a Character Web

Truby offers two models for thinking about how all of your characters are connected in your storytelling. His first "character web" model focuses on function in the story; the second focuses on archetypes. They are linked and both are useful, but we will discuss the latter here.

Truby's paradigm adapts Jung's categories slightly, but his archetypes are clear and their core functions are straightforward. You can also read his introductory description of archetypes in the Sage Spotlight on page 86. Following Jung's notion of the shadow, or the negative side of an archetype, Truby gives each one a benign or malign potential: The King might be an oppressor; the Mother might smother or guilt-trip; the Mentor might be overly rigid and didactic; the Warrior might despise the weak and prey on them. This is a useful reminder, and a first step away from thinking of these categories as static and predictable. I'll give a few simple examples shortly, but you can follow up with his book for the full discussion.

It's important to note also that the archetypes do not have to be rigidly gendered. The Mother can be a male and the Wise Old Man might be a woman or nonbinary person. Once again, when you are writing it is vital to remember that every King or Queen or Rebel is different and individual, even if they share common archetypal traits. Catch yourself when you begin to think in conventional terms and instead redirect your attention to what you believe this individual character *would* do in your story, rather than what it seems a generic character like that *should* do. Refocus on the individual details of your characters. Once again, your story's theme can help you, because every character must engage in some way with it. That begins to define their purpose in ways that will also inform how they inhabit their archetype.

In the list here, you'll find examples of each archetype.

THE KING OR FATHER

A wise leader or a tyrannical oppressor.

> King Arthur in *Excalibur* (1981), Washizu Taketoki in *Throne of Blood/Kumonosu-jō* (1957).

THE QUEEN OR MOTHER

A nurturing protector or an overbearing oppressor.

> Galadriel in the *Lord of the Rings* trilogy, Marion McPherson in *Lady Bird* (2017).

THE WISE OLD MAN OR MENTOR

Passes on knowledge. The mentor can push too far and too hard like bad teachers and football coaches do.

> Yoda in the *Star Wars* movies, Mary Poppins in *Mary Poppins* (1964).

THE WARRIOR

Enforces what is right or what is wrong.

> Brienne of Tarth from *Game of Thrones* (2011–2019), the T800 in *The Terminator*.

THE MAGICIAN OR SHAMAN

Brings balance and can control hidden forces or blow them up.

> Emma from Jane Austen's *Emma*, Saruman in *The Lord of the Rings*.

THE TRICKSTER

Uses trickery and persuasion to achieve their goals, for good or for ill.

Wichita in *Zombieland* (2009), Arya Stark in *Game of Thrones*.

THE ARTIST OR CLOWN

Defines excellence or uses humor to critique or creates artificial or even fascistic ideals of perfection.

Susan Cooper in *Spy* (2015), Amy in *Trainwreck* (2015).

THE LOVER

Uses care and sensuality to make others happy or dominate them.

Shakespeare's Juliet in *Romeo and Juliet*, Brandon in *Shame* (2011).

THE REBEL

Acts against oppressive systems or tries to overthrow good/democratic/ [insert values] order.

Jyn Erso in *Rogue One: A Star Wars Story* (2016), Clyde Barrow in *Bonnie and Clyde* (1967).

It is also worth noting that Truby argues that archetype-like functions can articulate the arc of change a goal-driven character goes through in the story. A character might start as one function and then change to another: Shakespeare's Macbeth begins the play as a Warrior or Leader, a loyal soldier to King Duncan, and then becomes a King, but in the negative form of a Tyrant, after he kills Duncan and takes the throne. Similarly, Truby suggests that Rick in *Casablanca* changes from Cynic to Participant, Oskar Schindler in *Schindler's List* (1993) changes from Adult to Leader, and so forth.

SAGE SPOTLIGHT:
John Truby on Archetypes

Here is John Truby's argument for archetypes, and his warning, which I fully endorse, about the danger of a poorly executed archetype web:

"Archetypes are fundamental psychological patterns within a person; they are roles a person may play in society, essential ways of interacting with others. Because they are basic to all human beings, they cross cultural boundaries and have universal appeal. Using archetypes as a basis for your characters can give them the appearance of weight very quickly, because each type expresses a fundamental pattern that the audience recognizes, and this same pattern is reflected both within the character and through interaction in the larger society. An archetype resonates deeply with an audience and creates very strong feelings in response. But it is a blunt tool in the writer's repertoire. Unless you give the archetype detail, it can become a stereotype."

—John Truby, *The Anatomy of Story: 22 Steps to Becoming a Master Storyteller*

A Hero's Journey

Vogler's approach to storytelling is steeped in the structure of myth, so of course he's drawn to archetypes. *The Writer's Journey* is deeply influenced not only by Jung, but also by the work of literary scholar Joseph Campbell. Campbell's ideas became influential in Hollywood in the 1970s after George Lucas and other young filmmakers championed his book, *The Hero with a Thousand Faces*. There, Campbell posits the concept of a "monomyth," as heroic stories from across cultures share common structural tropes.

Vogler's book updates and translates Campbell's work into the vernacular of Hollywood screenwriting, moving toward Jung to suggest that myths are "like the dreams of an entire culture, springing from the collective unconscious." What is appealing about Vogler's approach is the way he looks at archetypes as flexible character functions. In any story, an archetype can manifest in certain behaviors rather than being the constant and defining trait of a particular character. A character might behave like a Mentor at one point in a story without necessarily being defined or bound by that archetype throughout.

In *Clueless* (1995), the protagonist, Cher, gives a memorable speech on immigration in her high school debate class. Her analogies to party crashing are insane, yet somehow apt, and she ends with a truly great line, reminding her classmates ". . . that it does not say RSVP on the Statue of Liberty." Is Cher really a Mentor? She does have Mentor tendencies but, as a compulsive matchmaker trying to help everyone she meets, she's primarily a weird version of Truby's Lover, or Vogler's Hero (see page 88). Even so, her wacky Mentor-ing certainly resonates as she adopts that archetypal function at this point in the story.

The following are Vogler's most common archetypes. You'll see how they overlap with Truby's. I have used examples from *Star Wars: Episode IV – A New Hope*, because the movie's structure was strongly influenced by Campbell's writing.

Over the course of the original *Star Wars* trilogy, several characters change their primary archetype, in particular Han Solo, Darth Vader, and Princess Leia. It is important to note that some of the terms, like

Threshold Guardian, are chosen to fit into the beats of the structural model of mythic storytelling Vogler adapts from Campbell.

THE HERO

Luke Skywalker wants to be more than a moisture farmer.

THE MENTOR

Obi-Wan Kenobi wants to help Luke become a Jedi.

THRESHOLD GUARDIAN

Minor villains and obstacles. There are many options here, but remember those nasty guys in the cantina? Yeah, well they don't like you, either.

HERALD

R2-D2 brings Leia's message.

SHAPESHIFTER

Leia, because she takes on different roles and functions.

SHADOW

Darth Vader; he's the darkness in Luke's world.

ALLY

Chewbacca is the loyal friend (and occasional critic) to Han and others.

TRICKSTER

Han Solo. Just ask Greedo.

Vogler suggests that we can look at the archetypes as facets of the hero's personality, as well as story functions. That's because each archetype has a psychological as well as a dramatic function. According to Vogler, the Hero's psychological function is to represent the ego. The mythic hero's journey can be read as a search for wholeness and identity and, in psychological terms, the ego is at the center of this quest.

The Hero also has a number of important dramatic functions including audience identification—the Hero is our way into the story—and learning, or growth. Character change, as we know, is all-important for a goal-driven story: Luke is bored farming moisture on Tatooine and wishes he could be a space pilot. We identify with his desires and hope he gets his wish. And that brings us to the Herald.

To Vogler, the Herald represents the call to change. In psychological terms, this need for change manifests in a messenger of some kind—a dream, a person, or even an object with special meaning. In dramatic terms, the Herald is all about motivation. The Herald gets the protagonist moving in the story, or at least warns them that they are going to have to do something soon. R2-D2 brings Leia's message for Obi-Wan that Luke intercepts, right when he is looking for a way out of his life. Luke tries to find Obi-Wan to deliver the message and that gets him involved with the key personalities and events of the rebellion against the evil Empire.

HORROR ARCHETYPES FOR ANY GENRE

There are many screenwriting websites aimed at aspiring writers. Most cover exactly what you expect them to—a bit like this book, perhaps. Still, sometimes they surprise you, as with this little nugget from author John Bucher on the website LA Screenwriter. Bucher offers four rather specific archetypal figures that are coded for horror, but can also be used in any genre.

THE GHOST

Bucher's ghost archetype is someone from the past who haunts your protagonist, possibly making things complicated at just the wrong moment. In *A History of Violence* (2005), Carl Fogarty haunts the protagonist Tom Stall.

THE MONSTER

This is the most obvious of Bucher's suggestions, but lots of movies can use a monster to keep conflict ticking over. Like we saw with the dragon queen in *How to Train Your Dragon*, monsters are often obstacles rather than antagonists.

THE VAMPIRE

Vampires are parasites and they can turn up in any genre. Bucher offers the excellent example of Walter Keane, who takes credit for his wife's work in *Big Eyes* (2014).

THE FRANKENSTEIN

Frankensteins are innocent or harmless characters who are persecuted as monsters, like Boo Radley in *To Kill a Mockingbird*. As Bucher writes: "The point of the 'Frankenstein' archetype is to reveal shortcomings in the protagonist or the society they live in, not shortcomings in the 'Frankenstein.'"

In the Writers' Room:
AN ARCHETYPE EXERCISE

This exercise is about writing archetypes, not stereotypes. Pick an archetype from the many examples on the previous pages and address each of these four questions with a sentence.

1. What kind of character would I typically expect this archetype to produce?
2. How could my character have the same function in my story, but be unique and interesting?
3. How can my interpretation of my character's archetype make them a strong/interesting/entertaining character?
4. How can my interpretation of my character's archetype imply a weakness?

For example, we might pick a Mentor archetype and write the following four sentences:

1. I would expect a Mentor to be an old man who gives sage advice, possibly while scratching his long white beard.
2. This character is actually my protagonist's older sister, who teaches him how to play Ramones bass lines so he can audition for the punk band led by his crush.
3. She has mad musical skills and she has been through the local scene before, so she has contacts—and enemies—and can help her brother get in with the right people (if he'll let her).
4. She is arrogant and has little patience for anyone who isn't a fast learner, even her brother.

See what we did there? I had no idea who this character was before I started to write these sentences—I didn't even know she was a "she." Now I can see loads of story potential here: We are in the world of teen romance and high school punk bands, which makes that tired old trope more interesting. The brother/ sister relationship will have major tensions, but she's cooler than anyone ever had the right to be, so when the siblings are pulling together, who knows what they can achieve? Maybe they start their own band and the brother's crush is so impressed that she comes to them. Why isn't the sister in a band? Maybe she's a great bass player but she has performance anxiety or is pulling away from music after a fight with an old bandmate. And so, the spider diagram of inspiration begins to work.

Similarly, we might pick the Vampire archetype and write these four sentences:

1. This character is a terrifying undead creature who wants nothing more than to suck the lifeblood from my protagonist's veins.

2. This character is my protagonist's best friend, who borrows money all the time and hardly ever pays it back.

3. But that makes him very persuasive; he can always get his buddy to open his wallet—ah, so he's a vampire/trickster maybe . . .

4. On the other hand, maybe that's what gets him into trouble, because he also borrows from the wrong people and they break your knees if you don't pay up.

See how it works? This is another storyline that is writing itself, just because we thought creatively about

CONTINUED ►

an archetype for a single character. Yeah, it's not the most original idea in the world, but it leads to another, and then another ...

Now, what if both those characters are in the same movie? (I know, mind blown.)

Our protagonist—let's call him Joey—is an aspiring high school musician. He has a crush on the singer in a punk band (Kris) and wants to learn bass (because guitar is too hard and would take too long) to get in with her. His sister (Mags) is a great bass player and knows the scene. Problem: She's a hard-ass and will push him beyond his limits as a musician. Meanwhile, his best buddy (everyone calls him Poor Boy or P. B. for short) is a charming no-goodnik. He's always broke and pestering our protagonist for a loan. P. B. owes the wrong people, including the antagonist (Hilly), who happens to run the only punk club in town. Mags hates Hilly because he stiffed her on a performance fee back in the day. Hilly hates Mags because she got in his face about it in front of everyone. Now we have a setup for a story.

Here's a possible archetype breakdown for the major roles in this emerging movie with some choices or possible mid-story shifts:

Joey—Lover/Warrior

Kris—King/Lover

Mags—Mentor/Queen

Poor Boy—Vampire/Trickster

Hilly—King

Ideally you can use this exercise to give some depth or originality to characters in one of your own screenplays, but it works as an abstract thought exercise as well. Now it's your turn.

WRITE YOUR LOGLINE

Once you've thought through the characters and structure of your story, it's time to encapsulate those ideas in a logline. You have the nuts and bolts in place, and you're ready to start building (or rather, writing).

A logline is a very short statement that encapsulates your story concept and *sells your idea*. Typically, you use it in a meeting to help introduce or pitch your movie concept. Working out your movie's logline is also a great way of assessing your own idea and testing it out before you develop it further. In this chapter we are going to work on developing a great logline and use it to facilitate and discipline your screenwriting.

In short, if you have a good logline, you can write your screenplay, pitch it, and sell a movie.

WHAT IS A LOGLINE?

A logline should be a sentence—and certainly no more than two sentences—that helps your reader or listener "get" the concept of your movie. There will be more that you need to say as the meeting progresses, but everything that comes after your logline should make sense because it fits into the logic you have already established.

Here's an example of a logline that I put together for a well-known movie. Can you work out what it is?

> **"A man who can't create short-term memories has to find a way to remember clues in his hunt for his wife's killer."**

The answer is *Memento* (2000), written and directed by Christopher Nolan. If it wasn't too difficult to work out, it means the logline was effective (assuming you're already familiar with the movie).

Here's another one:

> **"An idealistic lawyer must defend an innocent black man accused of raping a white woman, even though his community demands a conviction."**

The answer is the classic Harper Lee novel that was turned into a movie, *To Kill a Mockingbird*.

As you can see from these examples, the logline doesn't tell you everything that happens in the movie. Instead, it sells the core concept and tells you enough to be able to understand how any additional information will fit with that concept. Your logline needs to grab people and leave them wanting more.

Why Do Loglines Matter?

A great logline can get your screenplay read and your movie made.

Regardless of how you develop a story, you will need to create a succinct and accurate way to describe it. This is for your own benefit, as well as for the benefit of future producers and audiences. Working out a logline is one way to start disciplining your thinking.

A logline gives you logical questions to answer about your concept as you develop it. "Does this idea for a relationship or a scene fit my logline?" If so, great. If not, that means you need to think a bit harder about that question—or rethink your logline. If the logline isn't quite right, the overall story probably needs tweaking, too. This is an important thought exercise to work through before you get too far along in your screenplay development.

What a Logline Is Not

We'll explore what makes a good logline in a moment, but to start, let's disentangle it from a related, but distinct, term: A logline is not a tagline.

Unlike a logline, a tagline is a marketing statement used on posters and ads once the movie is made. A logline is a selling statement you use to pitch a concept for a movie or to get someone interested in reading your screenplay. You might use a logline to open your pitch in a meeting with a producer, a development executive, an agent, or a manager. Taglines come much later.

Here are some examples of famous *tag*lines:

Bonnie and Clyde: "They're young, they're in love, and they kill people."
Mars Attacks! (1996): "Nice planet. We'll take it!"
Monsters, Inc. (2001): "We scare because we care."
Get Out: "Just because you're invited doesn't mean you're welcome."

Some of those are familiar, right? If you remembered them, the taglines were effective. What's more, they made you want to know more about the movie. In short, these taglines are great instances of marketing. But that's not your job. Your job is to persuade people to make the movie in the first place. If you're successful with your logline, the marketing department can thank you with their taglines down the road.

Your job is to write loglines, not taglines.

I'm emphasizing the difference before we get into what makes a great logline because the terms slip over each other in common usage, even though they mean something quite different in practice. If you Google "loglines," you will probably get more results that are actually taglines. When you do get loglines, they will likely be examples of how to write loglines, not authentic loglines used for any actual movie. This is because the logline for a movie is something that is typically lost after the pitch. It is part of the invisible development process that you won't know about unless you experience it yourself or you hear about it from friends in the business. What emerges in public, after the development process, is the tagline, not the logline.

WHAT MAKES A GREAT LOGLINE?

Remember how we established that a logline is designed to sell your story, not to tell it? The first step to selling is understanding that nobody will buy your concept if they don't get it.

Begin your logline creation by asking yourself this obvious but vital question: "What does somebody need to know about my movie concept in order to understand it?" Put as much of your answer into a coherent sentence or two as you can, and you have a working logline.

Your answer to the question may include a number of items, not all of which need to make their way into your logline. Here's the list:

- the protagonist(s)
- the antagonist(s)
- the genre
- the conflict
- the challenge
- the stakes
- the theme
- the twist
- the hook—*that one unique thing that makes your concept fly*
- the inciting incident

All of those categories are useful, but the hook is the big seller. The hook is the thing that piques your interest and makes you want to know more. In a genre movie, the hook is often about how you turn or twist the genre, or how you combine elements of more than one genre into a compelling hybrid form. In a character-driven movie, it often lies in the combination of a unique character and their goal or theme.

Character-driven movies are typically harder to write loglines for than plot-driven movies because the form of a logline tends to prioritize plot over story. This brings us to our next point.

Inciting Incident and Loglines

The inciting incident is often part of a useful logline. Let's look at some more simple, if silly, plot-driven science fiction loglines that might play off the inciting incident directly. Here's one off the top of my head: "When evil aliens kill her partner [inciting incident], tough Brooklyn beat cop Lauren Brown [protagonist] must battle her way to their home planet [challenge] to get her revenge [theme]." Loglines might also reveal genre. In this example, the listener can grasp it is a hybrid science fiction and revenge movie, but the logline didn't waste words telling us that because the other elements made it obvious.

Or how about we indulge in a science fiction romantic comedy heist movie? "When aliens abduct [inciting incident] bored Brooklyn accountant Jenny Yang [protagonist], she finds unexpected love and criminal adventure [hook] at the side of the dashing space captain [love interest] and their gang of interstellar jewel thieves." It's *Ocean's Eleven* (2001) meets *Desperately Seeking Susan* (1985) on the set of *Firefly*.

Silly stuff, of course, but in each case you see how the parts fit to tell you all you need to know to understand the basic concept of the movie. Don't be tempted to add more subclauses to your basic logline. (That's what your pitch meeting is for.) Keep the first statement short, sweet, and clear. The goal is to prevent your audience from thinking, "Wait, what?" Instead they should be asking, "What happens next?!"

Plot or Story?

In everyday conversations, we use the words "plot" and "story" interchangeably. In screenwriting, there are important distinctions, and we have already been using them in this book. It goes like this:

1. A movie has both a plot and a story (it also has subplots, as we learned earlier).

2. The plot is the events we see on-screen. People meet, talk, love, fight, chase each other around, and do all kinds of active things.

3. The story is the subtext. It is the deeper meaning that drives the plot; it's what we infer from watching the plot. The story is about why we talk, love, fight, etc., and what those surface actions mean for the characters who do them. It is the personal, emotional journey your protagonist makes in dealing with the theme of your movie.

Loglines tend to foreground plot over story because the screenwriter needs to provide enough plot-related facts in their opening sentence for the concept to make sense. That tends to push explanation of emotional arcs (which *drive* the plot) down to secondary statements in this particular context.

For example, this logline could work for the character-driven indie movie *Winter's Bone*: "In rural Missouri, a teenage girl [protagonist] risks violent retribution [stakes] by breaking the rules of her drug-cooking clan [conflict] to find her fugitive father [challenge] and save her family home [theme]." By dint of her age alone, this girl must be out of her depth. Also, the stakes couldn't be higher for her family. This sounds like great drama, even though we don't yet know how our young protagonist, Ree Dolly, will drive the movie.

Let's say this logline piques the attention of a producer or development executive and they want to know more. You could carry that part of the discussion forward by being ready to explain, with your next breath, that: "She is able to move the immovable by dint of her courage, intelligence, and sheer force of will." This sentence plays to her character and is an example of why developing a two-sentence logline can sometimes be a good idea.

Let's do one more for good measure. A basic logline for *Alien* might go like this: "The crew of a commercial spacecraft answers a distress signal, encountering a terrifying alien species. Once the creature is loose on their ship, they must fight for survival against the perfect killer."

The formula for this logline looks like this: ensemble protagonist + inciting incident + conflict + antagonist. The hook is that this monster-in-the-house movie is set on a spaceship. Is there more to say? Of course. In particular, we know nothing about the uniqueness of the alien yet, and that's huge. Does it give us every subplot? No. But do we "get" what action will take place, and how the movie will move forward? Yes.

Loglines and Genre

Unless your idea is truly experimental and non-narrative, in which case you are more likely to be writing an artist's statement in a grant application, it's important to be able to identify your genre or story type as you develop your logline. After all, in most cases you'll have to find a way to connect with audiences through a familiar lens (or set of lenses). Genres are all about that: audience connection.

Even if you don't think of your story in terms of a conventional genre—or even a clear hybrid—the way genre fandom works can help you look for a hook. When you are writing in a given genre, it's your job to deliver on what the audience expects *and* create something new. Genre fans expect their genre of choice—for example, a western, a horror film, a romantic comedy, a thriller—to be recognizable in some way. It needs to convey a certain western-ness, thriller-ness, etc. This familiarity gives us a level of comfort: "I know what this is and I like it." But if your script is too genre-conforming, it runs the risk of feeling unoriginal. To co-opt the language of cinema studies, your genre story needs to hit a good balance between repetition and difference. Your logline can foreground your innovative approach to genre, or not, as appropriate.

BREAKOUT STAR:
Noam Kroll

"The logline is truly an art form of its own. It's the one- or two-sentence summary of your film that not only conveys your premise, but also gives the reader emotional insight into the story as a whole. Loglines were used in the early days of Hollywood so producers could read a short explanation of a script (most often printed on the spine of the screenplay), allowing them to skip over uninteresting screenplays without even pulling them out from the shelf. While loglines today are no longer printed on the screenplays themselves, they effectively serve the exact same purpose—to efficiently represent the story and get the potential reader interested."

—Noam Kroll, writer-director of *Shadows on the Road* (2018)

We were discussing *Alien* as a genre hybrid earlier, so let's go into a little more detail. The logline can—and should—hint at the feeling we will get from experiencing the merging of science fiction and horror. This genre merger is key to the success of the concept and of the movie, so let's see how it works: When we watch *Alien*, the first scenes play as science fiction. We are on the spaceship when the crew is awakened from deep sleep; groggily, they figure out where they are and why they have been awakened early. That's a bit of a mystery, but we still feel securely in the realm of science fiction. For one thing, everything looks like sci-fi, with spaceships, space suits, alien planets, and so forth. As an exercise in story world creation, it presents with the science fiction-ness we seek out as genre fans. There's the repetition.

Later in the first act, the crew encounters the alien spaceship and its cargo of eggs, and here, the tone of the movie changes rapidly to horror. The ship itself is weird and scary with biological elements in its design. Uncanny eggs contain vicious alien "facehuggers," one of which attaches to the face of a crew member. From that moment on, the scares ramp up. There's the difference.

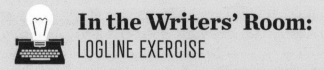

In the Writers' Room:
LOGLINE EXERCISE

After you work on this exercise a few times, you'll be able to pitch the movie you are writing or planning to write. It comes in three parts. You can use your own movie ideas or you can invent movie concepts for this exercise, which is repeatable as many times as you like—who knows, you might like one of your ideas enough to develop it for a new screenplay.

1. Invent a *protagonist*. Give them a job, a key personality trait, an attitude to the world, a need, or a goal. Optionally, you can decide on a genre here as well, or let it emerge as you develop the character and, thus, the concept.

2. Now you need *conflict*, which means an antagonist. It doesn't have to be a person. Winter could be an antagonist in a wilderness survival movie, for example. Ask yourself how your antagonist is a perfect foil for your protagonist.

3. Ask yourself, "What's at *stake*?" What will happen if the antagonist wins?

4. Optionally add a plot *twist* for high-concept fun.

5. Put at least one aspect of your answers to each of these questions into a sentence and you have a basic logline.

Kick-starting your logline: Remember my offhand comment: "It's *Ocean's Eleven* meets *Desperately Seeking Susan* on the set of *Firefly*"?

To be clear, an "X meets Y" shorthand is not a logline, but it is the way some movie people talk about story ideas. I wouldn't pitch this way because it's the height of cheese and it would make a bad impression in a meeting—especially if the people didn't know you well. (And I would certainly never open with that kind of statement, for the same reason, even if the discussion that followed might make use of this kind of shorthand.) But for some people, thinking in shorthand can be helpful when explaining about how a new idea relates to existing successful movies. This type of thought exercise might help you develop a hook or fine-tune an idea that isn't quite working yet.

OUTLINE YOUR SCREENPLAY

Now you're ready to take the next step in your movie writing, and that's to work out your story from first to last scene. In particular, we are going to focus on treatments and outlines, which both deal with the entire story of your movie. Note that treatments and outlines are different documents, written in very different styles and for different readerships.

This is important: While you might be tempted to launch straight into writing script pages, if you write a good outline first, you will have more fun when it comes to the screenplay and a better chance of finishing what you started. That's a promise.

WHY BOTHER WITH AN OUTLINE?

So, now you have a logline. Congratulations! That means you have a good grasp on the concept of your film, right? (If you don't, then maybe play around with the exercise in the last chapter a couple more times and get it nailed down.) In order to move into the outline stage, you'll need a strong concept like that to drive and discipline your development process.

With a concept that is working for you and a logline in hand, it's time to test them out by developing a short outline of the whole film. An outline is a summary of your entire story that breaks it into acts, beats, sequences, and scenes. It includes:

- the movie's title
- your logline
- a long synopsis

Your outline puts flesh on the bones of your logline. An outline tells you what happens in every scene of your movie; however, it does not answer every question that a development executive might have, because its primary purpose is not to persuade. That's what a treatment is for, and we'll give you examples of both shortly.

Having said that, a good outline will give you the confidence that you have a real story to develop because it gives you enough information to keep on track as you write. You can go back to your outline as you write, expanding it and filling in minor gaps as the act of writing inspires you. Let's say you write a scene, and it brings into focus something that happens later in the story. Great. Add that new insight to your outline.

Now, here's where you might get different advice on how to proceed. Some screenwriters and screenwriting teachers feel strongly that you need to have everything nailed down in your outline—every scene, even some dialogue—before you start writing screenplay pages. Others—myself included—believe that while it is important to "break your story" (Hollywood jargon for "work out its basic structure"), over-preparation can be harmful to the creative process. When you are just starting out, it may be hard for you to conceptualize your entire story at that level of precision. You shouldn't feel concerned if you are unable to place every scene of your first screenplay right out the gate. Welcome to screenwriting; some aspects do get easier with experience.

Regardless of your approach, then, the goal of an outline is to work out how your story develops and resolves scene by scene. The more you know before you start writing actual scenes, the easier the draft will be. Let's pause for a moment to clarify some common terms that relate to an outline and are easy to mix up.

Outlines and Treatments—What's the Difference?

You might have heard these words bandied about and, in common usage, they seem to slip over each other and share meanings. Once again, it's important to understand their unique meanings in the context of screenwriting. In short, writers use outlines to prepare to write their scripts; writers use treatments to get employed and bring those scripts to fruition.

Outlines

Outlines are simple prose documents that writers create for their own use. An outline is where you structure the details of your story. In an outline, you lay out the scenes that drive and contain your theme, your acts, your beats, and your arcs until you have a complete framework for the script you are going to write. Full outlines are straightforward documents that offer you, the writer, utility. In your outlines, you put down information and ideas for your scenes so that you have something practical to reference when you are writing them into your script. Outlines can include sample dialogue and even some fully drafted scenes, but usually they offer a clear note for each scene, explaining who is doing what and the outcome.

An outline is essential for story development, and it is a supportive tool for creating a screenplay. However, you may also need to develop a range of targeted documents, all of which emphasize different aspects of your story, only for different audiences. Every grant-awarding organization has its own mission statement and goals; if funding is on your mind, research them and write a version of your story as a treatment to appeal to this target organization. Your story won't change, but the angle of your pitch likely will.

There are no hard and fast rules for writing an outline. The point is that it be useful for you as you sit down to write your screenplay. It makes sense to organize your outline according to the model of storytelling you plan to use. For example, if you are working within the three-act paradigm, then you will split your story into three acts. A five-act structure, naturally, would have five acts.

SAGE SPOTLIGHT:
JOHN AUGUST'S OUTLINE

Here's a very brief, sequence-driven outline by screen-writer John August for the opening of his screenplay *Big Fish* (2003). He doesn't outline every scene, but rather works from a group of scenes that accomplish particular story tasks. Most outlines go scene by scene, but this sequence version works as well.

BIG FISH SEQUENCE OUTLINE 3/31/00

SEQ. 01 – PAGES 1–6 THE CATFISH
Edward tells the same big fish story throughout Will's life, finishing at Will's wedding. Will and Edward have an argument.

SEQ. 02 – PAGES 6–8 THOSE THREE YEARS
The next three years pass. Will's voice-over explains how he and his father communicated indirectly. Edward swims; Will and Josephine check on the health of their unborn child.

SEQ. 03 – PAGES 8–11 THE DAY
MY FATHER WAS BORN
Will tells the story of the day his father was born, the day it finally rained in Ashland.

SEQ. 04 – PAGES 11–14 WILL GETS THE PHONE CALL
Will gets word that his father's condition has worsened. He and Josephine board a plane for the States.

Treatments

A treatment is a *selling* document. Treatments are designed to be read and used by the executives, producers, and agents who will eventually buy and sell the movie project. You're writing the treatment for people who will decide whether it is worth paying you for a full screenplay draft. For this reason, your treatment will be written in the prose equivalent of master screen format.

A treatment contains much of the same information as an outline, but it is written in a more dynamic and compelling style. You are writing to show your readers that your story contains everything they could possibly want in a successful movie. (You can find an example of this style of writing in the Sage Spotlight on Terry Rossio, on page 110.)

One way to position your treatment is to write it in the tone of the movie. For example, a comedy treatment should anticipate that humor on the screen by being funny in both tone and content. Typically, a treatment includes more detail on film style and characters, relationships and motivations. There is a real art to treatment writing; the idea is to get your readers excited about your story through your prose.

WHY OUTLINE RESEARCH MATTERS

Screenplay research is always your friend. Well, until it isn't. It's great until you have done so much research that you can't see the forest for the trees.

As a rule of thumb, assume that you need to know more than your audience does. Not everything you learn from research will end up directly referenced in your movie. However, it will *inform* everything you include in your screenplay, and what we see on screen. If your characters have a certain profession, or set of religious beliefs, or political philosophy, you need to understand that. You need to understand the setting of your story, and how that might influence your characters' behavior. Bottom line: Do the legwork to know your story world.

SAGE SPOTLIGHT:
TERRY ROSSIO'S TREATMENT

Here's the opening of a treatment (not an outline) for
The Mask of Zorro (1998, treatment written in 1994) from
screenwriter Terry Rossio. Note how the dramatic prose
sells the mysterious nature of the movie's hero: Zorro
is "a black apparition in the moonlight" who the young
brothers watch "in wonderment."

"The opening sequence is told
through the eyes of two young
brothers, ALEJANDRO and JOAQUIN
MURIETTA. It takes place in Alta
California, 1822. Mexico is about
to win its independence. The Spanish Viceroy of California, MONTERO,
realizes his time is up. He has
ordered the execution of all political prisoners. The boys sneak
into the town square to watch
the hangings.

But Montero is foiled again by
ZORRO, who sails in and frees
the prisoners. Completely heroic,
a black apparition in the moonlight, Alejandro and Joaquin watch
him in wonderment. But Montero was
counting on Zorro's arrival; more
soldiers wait in ambush. Zorro is
unaware of the trap."

A BRIEF LOOK AT ADAPTATION

Adaptation is another big topic, and worthy of a book of its own. We'll just introduce it here and offer you a list of questions to consider if you're thinking about adapting a property from another medium into a screenplay.

Do you have the legal right to do it? First and foremost, if you don't own the copyright, have explicit (written) legal permission to sell the resulting screenplay, or you are not being employed to write the adaptation—don't do it. It's a waste of your time and nobody will read your script, for legal reasons. Incidentally, if you want to explore the possibility of getting the legal permission to adapt a book, or another intellectual property, you should contact the publisher and ask who owns the derivative rights for movie adaptation.

Is there a movie there? Assuming you do control the property or have permission to adapt it, ask yourself: How is this story cinematic? First and foremost, cinema is a visual medium—I know, who'd have thought, right? But that's important once again, because not all novels (for example) are easy to make visual. You need to have a plan to deal with the medium-specific aspects of whatever story you want to tell.

What are the particular challenges of your source medium? To take one example, comic books and graphic novels tell visual stories, but in a particular way. The story of a comic book carries an implied reading track that works from panel to panel and page to page. The visual power of a comic book lies in art that is static, even if it feels dynamic when we read around the page. Each panel is its own image, but the creative geometries of a comic book page are also laid out for you to appreciate as another level of visual storytelling. There's a reason why very few comic book movie adaptations actually engage with the comic book-ness of the original and just tell its story without investing in the form. The stylized and hard-boiled *Sin City* would be a notable exception.

The story will have its own thematic symbolism already written in, regardless of the medium from which you are adapting. Sometimes it's subtle, but often there is a rich well of imagery for you to draw from.

Even the most plot-driven novels take time to establish location, period, and so forth. In the end, the task of the adapter is to remain true to the source and its medium, while not being overly beholden to it.

In whatever way you approach an adaptation, you will need to break the story and develop an outline as with any other screenplay. One way of approaching it is to outline the source "as is" and then begin to cut and add as your interpretation drives you. This can lead to more literal and traditional adaptations, of course, because it is the structure of the source rather than your interpretation that is driving the outline from the start, but it can at least help you to clarify the story structure of the original. You can then step back and consider where to go next.

The same is true of any outline, as a matter of fact. Once you have a version of your story outlined, you have an entire movie in shorthand, on a few pages. This is an incredibly helpful resource, not just to drive your script writing in the immediate future, but to assess your story and give you the clarity to rethink it and develop it further before you commit to screenplay form. In other words, what this chapter has given you is a way forward to the next stage of writing your screenplay. And sometimes the greatest value in outlining is to expose the faults in your thinking and help you correct them.

BREAKOUT STAR:
Taika Waititi

In *Jojo Rabbit*, writer/director Taika Waititi takes the enormous risk of setting a comedy in Nazi Germany during the Second World War. What's more, he embodies Adolf Hitler as the imaginary friend of a young boy who hopes to prove himself worthy to his *Führer* by becoming a "good" Nazi as a member of the Hitler Youth.

Waititi gets away with it for a number of reasons, including adopting a style of storytelling that shifts fluidly and eloquently to accommodate tragedy. But the movie also works because it is grounded in just enough period realism that we have to take the comic tone seriously. The comedy is propped up by the feel (if not the obsessive accuracy) of period. It is accurate enough for us to experience the story as pathos. In other words, it takes its setting and its young protagonist seriously enough that we are never allowed to easily dismiss the content. *Jojo Rabbit* wears its period research lightly, but never lets us forget what is underpinning the drama.

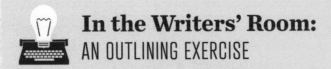

In the Writers' Room:
AN OUTLINING EXERCISE

The real exercise here is to outline your movie's story. If you have been following through with the guidelines and exercises in this book, you should be ready, so go to it!

If you need a little more thought, this preparatory exercise is intended to help you work toward your story's structure from another angle.

Name and describe characters who embody most or all of the following dramatic functions in your story, giving them each a different attitude to your theme: *protagonist, antagonist, helper, blocker, distracter, rival, advisor*. In other words, populate your story with characters who are invested in its theme. Some may share the same or similar attitudes.

As before, to complete this exercise you'll need to know the answers to the following:

- Who is your protagonist?
- What do they want in the plot (a practical resolution)?
- What do they need in the story (a linked emotional resolution)?
- Who wants to stop them and why (your antagonist)?
- What is your genre, or your genres?
- What is your theme?

Most of the answers to these questions should at least be implied in your logline. To complete this exercise, you'll revisit your theme. All the other pieces of key information will inform your choices as we go forward.

1. Remember, every key character in your movie should have an attitude to, and/or a role that plays into your theme. The collision of their attitudes and roles creates conflict. Conflict = drama.
2. Each thematic relationship, such as the one between your protagonist and your antagonist, is a strand of your plot.

Now you know how to play out your plot and story in terms of characters and theme. That's the core of mainstream and much indie storytelling.

TELL A VISUAL STORY

No matter how good your writing is, no matter how elegant or dynamic your descriptions are on the page, as a screenwriter your words are designed to transcend the page. Your script (if all goes as planned) will be made into a movie.

This is one of the key differences between screenwriting and writing in any other medium. Words will become images—pictures in motion—and your task is to facilitate that transformation by anticipating the visual in prose. Your writing should communicate how the scenes shot from your script have the potential to be cinematic. You will find that reading a good screenplay is a remarkably visual experience, only all the images are projected in your mind.

The trick is to develop a writing style that helps your reader see the film come to life from your script. We're going to look at some examples in depth but, as you're working on your screenplay, ask yourself:

- How does the drama flow through my scenes?
- What am I paying attention to now—and now?

FORMATTING AS BACKBONE

Way back in Rule 1, you learned about writing action descriptions. We talked about master scene format, using white space, and thinking of each key moment in your scene as a separate thought-image. We also talked about how sometimes the conventions of grammar and syntax don't apply when you are trying to evoke a sense of drama, movement, or tension. You remember all of that, right? Good. Here, we are going to work these ideas through case studies to see how successful screenwriters evoke the visual in their prose.

Learning from the Pros

Let's start with a simple scene, taken from the opening of Damien Chazelle's script for *La La Land* (2016). Note how the script is written in the present tense, which is standard practice in a professional screenplay. The idea is to give the reader the impression that everything that unfolds in your script is happening ... now!

```
1 EXT. 101 FREEWAY - DAY

Cars are at a standstill. It's a horrific
traffic jam.

Morning rush hour. Sun beating down,
asphalt shimmering in the heat. The
blown-out downtown L.A. skyline hovers in
the distance.

We DRIFT past more CARS. Hear one snippet
of audio after another...

One driver taps his steering wheel to PROG
ROCK. Another sings to OPERA. A third raps
along to a HIP-HOP track. We move from
a RADIO INTERVIEW to a FRENCH BALLAD to
TECHNO, until finally we begin to hear...
```

```
... a new, original piece of music...
[ANOTHER DAY OF SUN]
```

Note how Chazelle splits his description into bite-size chunks separated by white space. We absorb an image, or a linked cluster of images, and then we move on. It's like each short paragraph represents a shot, a moment of dramatic focus, or a very short sequence of shots, only he doesn't write them as shots, he writes them as images. In our minds, we put them together as a sequence. If he draws our attention to something small, we might imagine it in close up. If he describes the panorama, we "see" that in our minds as a wide shot.

Chazelle implies a camera move, but doesn't call it as such: "We DRIFT past more CARS . . ." It's a tracking shot, we get that, but drifting gives us the feeling of the technique—movement, speed—without specifying it. It keeps us in the story. This way, the images flow in our heads as we go from car to car, person to person. The script identifies them by sound—through their music choices, not their physical description—until finally the tune that will be the musical number for this sequence emerges from the mix.

This is simple, elegant screenwriting. It isn't flashy or in your face, but it brings us along on a journey through the cars in a way that feels natural. We aren't thinking about the techniques of movie production, just the flow of sound and image that his words create in our minds.

BREAKOUT STAR:
Damien Chazelle
on Writing Musicals

Chazelle, writer/director of **Whiplash** (2014) and **La La Land** talks to Ramona Zacharias of **Creative Screenwriting** about the hybrid nature of the musical:

"It's part of what I love about the musical as a genre in the first place. It's not realism, but it's also not pure fantasy. It's a genre that allows you to truly blend the two. And it's this kind of other world where emotion overrides everything, and if you feel a certain way, the world becomes a certain way. That's a very beautiful idea to me. It's a very hopeful idea, but it also can be a very sad idea because there always is this return to reality. I've always found some of the musicals that people think of as the happiest movies ever made to be somewhat heartbreaking as well. I think in the great musicals there is often this kind of sadness underneath. It's a wish fulfillment thing. Characters are trying to make the world into something that maybe it's not, into a more idealized vision of the world. There's a real poetry in that struggle, and sometimes that failure. I wanted to indulge in that kind of fantasy-making in this movie, and really push this aspect as far as I could. To literally have our characters waltz in outer space. But I also wanted to push the gritty reality as far as possible, even if that meant sitting at a dinner table with them for seven pages—seven minutes of screen time—watching them bicker in a very uncomfortable, claustrophobic sort of moment. The movie had to somehow fit both of those things."

Now, for contrast, let's read an extract from a draft of Tony Gilroy's screenplay for the thriller *The Bourne Identity* (2002). This shows a more dynamic and aggressive use of prose, as befits the opening of a thriller. The scene we'll read takes place near the start of the movie, when Jason Bourne has been saved from the ocean on the edge of death. On the fishing boat, the crew try to treat his wounds. (Gilroy uses double hyphens in his slugline below. Nowadays this is a relatively uncommon and somewhat old-fashioned formatting choice, but it's still technically acceptable.)

```
INT. FISHING BOAT BUNK ROOM - DAWN -
TIME CUTS

Transformed into a makeshift operating
room. A light swings overhead. THE MAN
layed out across the table. Sounds --
groans -- words -- snatches of them --
all in different languages.

GIANCARLO playing doctor in a greasy
kitchen apron. Cutting away the clothes.
Turning THE MAN on his side. Two bullet
wounds in the back. Probing them,
judging them.

Now -- GIANCARLO with a flashlight in his
teeth -- TINK -- TINK -- TINK -- bullet
fragments falling into a washed-out
olive jar.

Now -- something catching GIANCARLO'S
EYE -- A SCAR ON THE MAN'S HIP -- another
fragment -- exacto knife cutting in --
tweezers extracting A SMALL PLASTIC
TUBE, not a bullet at all, and as it
comes free --
```

```
THE MAN'S HAND SLAMS down onto GIANCARLO'S
and we SMASH CUT

INTO A --

FIRST PERSON POV -- we are staring up at --

                    GIANCARLO
          You're awake. Can you hear me?
```

This scene condenses time—hence "TIME CUTS" in the slugline—in order to highlight the important story information revealed by Bourne's treatment. Specifically, we learn that Bourne has bullet wounds, and that he has a small device or capsule implanted sub-dermally. These facts are solid expositional clues as to his job.

As you read through this extract, notice how Gilroy draws our attention from image to image all the way through. Once again, these are all implied shots or moments of cinematic focus. The finished movie scene uses a lot of closeups: a knife cutting through clothing and into skin; tweezers extracting bullet fragments, and so forth. With repeated use of the word "Now . . ." he orients us to the moment onscreen and guides our focus around the space and time of the action so that we see it as a sequence of discrete images. However, Gilroy never actually calls a shot until Bourne wakes up and we take his point of view: "FIRST PERSON POV . . ."

Gilroy's writing is also frequently punctuated by double hyphens, a common stylistic choice for dynamic and action scene writing. The effect of these punctuations is to break the continuity of grammar and syntax, drawing us from image to image, just as the finished scene will use jumps in its editing strategy to make time cuts. Each double hyphen flashes us forward -- next moment -- next image -- no need for syntax. Kinesis trumps coherence. It wouldn't work in *La La Land,* but it works great in *The Bourne Identity.*

Note how Gilroy uses onomatopoeia to punctuate the visual with implied sound. As the bullet fragments fall into the olive jar (a tray in the final film) they go "TINK -- TINK -- TINK . . ." That's a genre noise. That bullet TINK encapsulates something deeply embedded in our fandom because we know that noise from other thrillers and police procedurals. Every treatment and autopsy scene has its variant on the TINK. It is eloquent, evocative, familiar, and helps to bind our attention through recognition. Remember how we discussed genres being a combination of repetition and difference? That idea works at every level from big story elements to tiny sound effects. We don't know who Jason Bourne is, yet, but -- TINK -- we are in a thriller, and off we go.

It's important not to directly copy what Chazelle and Gilroy do. These are just two examples of screenwriting style that fit the vision for *their* movies. There are as many ways to write a scene as there are writers. Instead, ask yourself what the writers are trying to achieve with their different styles for scenes in very different genres. Then, ask how it affects the way you read and absorb each scene. It is the intention of a screenwriter's style that's important, not whether he or she happens to use ellipses or double hyphenation.

FROM THE INSIDE, OUT

A different sort of problem is how to communicate interiority—internal dialogue, emotions, the complexity of human thought and feelings—on the page. The short answer: People say revealing things (even if they are untrue) and people *do* revealing things. We can also infer interiority from context. For example, if we have seen in a previous scene that a character has experienced something unpleasant—they've suffered a loss or an injury, or they have witnessed something terrible—then we can infer emotional meaning from their reactions later in the script.

Similarly, as a writer, while you should not tell us directly what somebody is feeling when we have no context, you can indicate it with behavioral action. If your protagonist witnessed her brother's death in the hospital in one scene and is at home crying in the next, the audience will understand the connection across the cut; in this case, it would be appropriate to write an action instruction such as "Josephine grieves."

That's not a cheat, it is an obvious statement in the context of the story. A cheat would be an instruction in your opening scene: "Josephine grieves for the death of Sir Reginaldo III, her boyfriend's parrot who was killed by the neighbor's cat, and Josephine believes if only she hadn't left the door open it wouldn't have happened." I mean, how do we see that? Plus, it's the opening scene, so we have no context.

Experienced and talented writers find ways to get right up to the line with emotional instruction, as in this scene from Sofia Coppola's screenplay for *Lost in Translation* (2003).

```
INT. HOTEL RESTAURANT - DAY

They sit in the bright light. She squints
and drinks a Bloody Mary. Bob is distant.

She looks across at two middle-aged MID-
WESTERN WOMEN talking about plastic
surgery, you can't hear them, but can
tell as they gesture and one pulls her
eye lids up.

Charlotte looks at another table by the
elaborate buffet and sees the redhead
Singer having breakfast with the rest
of Sausalito.

                CHARLOTTE
          (trying to make it light)
     Hey look, it's Sausalito.

                BOB
     I see them every morning.
```

```
They don't know what to say. Somehow it's
too intimate having breakfast. She eats
her breakfast aware of her every movement.

C.U. - her POV of soft scrambled eggs.
```

Let's consider two statements.

1. "Bob is distant." This is general enough that the script gets away with it. It indicates a behavior more than a specific emotion.

2. "They don't know what to say. Somehow, it's too intimate having breakfast. She eats her breakfast aware of her every movement." Following the lead from "Bob is distant," Coppola could simply have written something such as, "It's awkward," and we would have understood the moment, albeit in a dull and prosaic fashion. However, in the context of the wider story which details Bob and Charlotte's friendship-that-never-quite-develops-into-something-more-but-in-another-life-perhaps-it-could-have, this statement speaks to a shared sense of the weight of their not-relationship.

SCENE ALCHEMY

As we discussed in rule 1, a screenplay scene happens in one time and place. If either the time or the location changes, then the scene should change with it.

As we have noted, scenes in Hollywood movies usually don't run to more than a couple of pages, and they infrequently last longer than two minutes on screen. A five-page scene would be the rare exception and a scene of this length would be reserved for a very special dramatic purpose. In less mainstream forms of cinematic storytelling, such as dialogue-heavy character-driven movies, scenes may average more pages/minutes, but that is by no means the rule.

The Rules of Purpose

Syd Field reminds us that scenes have two purposes. They should reveal character, or they should move the story forward. If they do neither, then the scene either needs rewriting or to be cut from your script. Remember that every page of your screenplay costs money to produce. Nobody wants to waste that money on scenes that have no real purpose. Besides, your professional colleagues will spot useless flab in your writing immediately.

A common example of a pointless scene that I find in student scripts is the generic friends-bantering scene. The writer thinks they are revealing character, but nothing changes, nothing develops. We learn nothing important (other than we don't trust your writing anymore).

Scenes are the basic building blocks of your storytelling. Some are simple, containing one action or a straightforward intention that moves the story forward. This can be a good thing because if every scene is deep and complex, your audience never gets a break. Sometimes, you just show us an image that the story context marks as poignant or revelatory. Other times, you are controlling the pace and giving us a breather—a chance to anticipate the upcoming action (but still writing a scene with purpose!).

In short, don't be frightened of letting some of your scenes be eloquently simple. We will appreciate them playing in the mix with more complex ones.

SCENE BEATS

Like full movie stories, complex scenes have their own internal structure of "beats." These are moments when the drama advances or the focus shifts in a meaningful way. Scene beats are important structural events that change the dynamic of character interactions and advance the plot. They are also important because actors and directors look for scene beats to guide them in their rehearsals and in performance.

Here's a classic example from the romantic gangster movie *Bonnie and Clyde*, written by David Newman & Robert Benton. Clyde meets Bonnie and starts to flirt with her. The scene turns when she asks him why he's looking for work and he replies that he was in prison. Now she has a big decision to make. Do I keep talking to this handsome ex-convict or get the hell away from him? In this case we kind of know the answer before she does—after all, the movie isn't titled *The Next Girl He Meets on the Street and Clyde*. And yet the outcome of the scene—and the rest of the movie—depends on what Bonnie does with that information. It depends on how she responds to that beat.

```
It is a hot Texas afternoon, all white
light and glare. As they walk the block to
town in this scene, their manner of mutual
impudence is still pervading.

                    CLYDE
          Goin' to work, huh? What do you do?


                    BONNIE
          None of your business.


                    CLYDE
              (pretending to give
               it serious thought)
          I bet you're a... movie star!
                    (thinks)
          No... A lady mechanic?... No...
          A maid?--


                    BONNIE
            (really offended by that)
          What do you think I am?
```

                    CLYDE
              (right on the nose)
A waitress.

                    BONNIE
          (slightly startled by his
           accuracy, anxious to get
             back now that he is
            temporarily one-up)
What line of work are you in? When
you're not stealin' cars?

                    CLYDE
              (mysteriously)
I tell you, I'm lookin' for suitable
employment right at the moment.

                    BONNIE
What did you do before?

                    CLYDE
         (coolly, knowing its effect)
I was in State Prison.

Boom! There's the scene beat, and . . .

                    BONNIE
              (sarcastically)
My, my, the things that turn up in the
driveway these days.

And off we go.

If scenes don't have a properly developed beat structure, then they
feel static. Robert McKee offers a useful shorthand by giving scenes a

polarity and then reversing it. A scene that begins on a positive note for the protagonist turns, on a beat, toward the negative. In other words, something bad happens, or vice versa. In the example above, Clyde's admission certainly turns the scene. Maybe the fact that it turns it from – to + for Bonnie, rather than the other way around, tells us a great deal about her and what she's searching for in life and love.

Objectives and Tactics

As you know, actors and directors will use your screenplay in their work. Writers need to think clearly about how their characters behave in scenes and how their work will be used by other professionals. The two key terms that relate to this writing-acting relationship are objectives and tactics.

Every significant character in a scene should have an objective. They come into the scene wanting something (a ham sandwich, a divorce), or they develop an objective as soon as a major plot or story event happens to them. It could be something simple and plot driven or something more subtle or complex. Actors read your script to set up their objectives and then they devise one or more tactics that their character will use to get what they want. If I want a piece of information from someone, I could *flirt* with them, *bully* them, *cajole* them, *reason* with them, and so on. All those options are potential tactics for an actor, and the way you write your scene will influence the way it is played. You need to think about your screenplay from the actors' point of view—and how objectives and tactics will emerge from the situation and dialogue—and voilà!—scene beats.

SAGE SPOTLIGHT:
John August on Writing Scenes

A-list screenwriter John August offers six questions to ask yourself and four tasks or exercises for when you are writing a scene. They are all important and worth following.

1. What needs to happen in this scene?
2. What would happen if this scene got omitted?
3. Who needs to be in the scene?
4. Where could the scene take place?
5. What's the most surprising thing that could happen in the scene?
6. Is this a long scene or a short scene?
7. Brainstorm three different ways it could begin.
8. Play it on the screen in your head.
9. Write a scribble version. (It's your outline: Get from start to finish in note form.)
10. Write the full scene.

A New Kind of Magic

Even in the farthest reaches of indie-land, scenes are still scenes. The rules of purpose—advancing plot and developing character—apply no matter what kind of story you're telling, although the terms of purpose might shift as your definition of story and storytelling diverges from the mainstream.

The options for writing good scenes are almost endless, regardless of who your intended audience is. Rather than making a vain attempt to encapsulate this huge range of choices in a few paragraphs, I'm going to offer a single example.

Here's a scene from the first draft of Scott Neustadter & Michael H. Weber's screenplay for *500 Days of Summer* that takes place the morning after our protagonist, Tom, first sleeps with his new love, the eponymous Summer. It uses tropes from fantasy, musicals, and even Disney-style animation to access Tom's feelings of joy. It's a sweet and funny scene—funny in part because these tropes are simultaneously out of place in a romantic drama and entirely appropriate, given how we understand the development of Tom's feelings. The story has earned its hyperbole. This is the only scene in the movie that works like this, but that's why it lands so well.

```
EXT. STREET - MORNING

It's the greatest morning of all time!

Tom walks down the street. Or, more accu-
rately, Tom struts down the street. He's
pointing at people as he passes, winking,
doing a little shuffle. He is the man.
He checks out his reflection in a window.
A YOUNG PAUL NEWMAN stares back.
```

People wave as he passes, they clap, they give him thumbs up. A parade forms behind him. The POSTMAN, a POLICE OFFICER, the HOT DOG VENDOR, RONALD MCDONALD and MAYOR MCCHEESE, everybody loves Tom today. HALL and OATES themselves walk with Tom singing the song.

Cars stop at crosswalks to let Tom go by. The DRIVERS also pump their fists in celebration of Tom's achievement last night. He walks on, the man. We notice the sidewalk lights up every time he touches the pavement like in "Billie Jean".

CARTOON BIRDS fly onto Tom's shoulder. He smiles and winks at them.

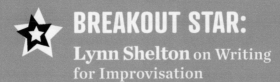

BREAKOUT STAR:

Lynn Shelton on Writing for Improvisation

In an interview with Slate's L.V. Anderson, the late writer/director Lynn Shelton discussed different approaches to preparing scenes and performances in her movies *Humpday* (2009) and *Your Sister's Sister* (2011):

"So many people have said this, but it's true: 95 percent of what I do as a director is casting and getting people who can bear the load of what you're asking them to do and creating this emotionally safe environment. With *Humpday*, it was a ten-page outline with no dialogue written at all. The structure was in place, I knew what I needed to take place in every scene—I wasn't just making it up as I went along. Then how the scenes got there is I just turned the cameras on and let the actors find their way. And ultimately the final draft is written in the edit room. You could have made 150 different movies out of the footage we shot, because there are so many different choices that they give me in terms of the beats and how it unfolds. But in the case of *Your Sister's Sister*, I actually had about seventy pages of dialogue written out, because I didn't have two veteran improvisers—I had one veteran improviser and two actors who were not used to working this way, and so I wanted them to have a sort of jumping-off point. A security blanket, if you will. So if they liked a line, they could feel free to use it. But I didn't want them to hold the lines too closely or hold even to the structure of the way the scene was going."

In the Writers' Room:
SCENE EXERCISE

Here's a short exercise in scene writing. You are going to write a scene of about three pages. Don't go over this limit if you can avoid it, but if your first draft is longer, that's fine. Just go back and see what dead wood you can cut. (I'm sorry to tell you this, but there's always dead wood.)

Here are the guidelines:

1. You have two characters, and each wants something from the other. That "something" could be an object, some information, an apology, an emotional connection of some kind, or something else that you decide.

2. Your characters know each other well.

3. Ask yourself how they would approach the challenge of getting what they want, not in the abstract but from the other character who they know. What kind of persuasion would work on them?

4. Give yourself three scene beats to develop the argument or discussion.

5. Make sure your scene turns for at least one of the characters from + to − or from − to +.

6. In the end, somebody wins. Maybe they both do. Maybe winning means no longer wanting the thing you came in wanting.

7. You cannot use action or violence. There will be no gunplay or car chases. The winner must succeed through dialogue alone.

MAP YOUR SEQUENCE

We have spent some time thinking about individual scenes, but scenes often work in combination in order to achieve a story goal. The power of sequences is that they build and reinforce your storytelling in ways that individual scenes cannot.

In this chapter we will consider this power, and the power of the story beat. This will lead us to discuss the challenge of pacing within and between all the beats of your story.

WHAT IS A SEQUENCE?

To be clear, at its most simple, a sequence is a group of scenes that combine to achieve one or more discrete storytelling goals. Sequences are usually connected on the basis of time and/or location, which give them dramatic unity. There is another context in which screenwriters talk about sequences, and that's when we break down our movies into story chunks or beats to plan them out. Sometimes this is called sequencing a movie. We will talk about both contexts in this rule, starting by asking the simple and obvious question: How does a sequence work?

Let's consider a classic, straightforward plot-driven sequence. A team of British commandos is scaling a cliff to attack the Nazi flak battery at the top. Now, you could achieve that in a couple of shots: commandos climb; oblivious guard at the top; commandos reach the top and attack him. You could also put together a much more dramatic sequence whereby we cut between different climbing teams (different locations on the same cliff, so there are scene changes) and the Germans on top of the cliff ranging in on the stream of aircraft carrying paratroops for D-Day. If our plucky commandos don't do their job, there will be hell to pay.

The "right" way to tell that part of your story depends on how you have set it up. Let's consider two ways of thinking about it. On the one hand, you might want to save your pages for the battle to come. These guys are commandos, so of course they can scale a cliff. We don't need to waste pages or screen time on it. On the other hand, maybe we have followed this group through their commando training. Private Jones is a bit of a klutz and the others worry that he will be a liability on the climb. Does he fall? Does he make it easily? Does he end up saving the guy who aced the climbing training? That may pay off serious character development, in the terms of the story. The same applies to the other characters. They are in danger and we care about them, so of course we want to see what happens in more detail. But maybe one of the commandos is a traitor—think of the action thriller *Where Eagles Dare* (1968). Do we know this, or is it a surprise? Are we waiting to see how that traitor will alert the guards? Is there a fight on the climbing ropes to stop him from yelling out? Who knows, but this version of the story puts a lot more weight [sic] on the climb. Either way, they contribute to or contain story beats.

SEQUENCES AND BEATS

There is often a difference between where a beat starts and where it lands (or pays off). In the example we used previously from *The World's End*, Gary King tells the story of the great unfinished pub crawl of his youth. Later, he is inspired to finish it, and that's where the beat lands. However, it starts at the beginning of his story: We need to hear the story, and then see him in his current circumstances in the AA meeting, to understand Gary's motivation. This beat sequence includes the narrated flashback, the catch-up scene at the meeting, and the moment of inspiration. Taken together this sequence is, in itself, a story beat. But some beats play longer than others. In longer story beats, we may need two or more sequences to do the work of significantly advancing the story, such as when we need to see something from multiple perspectives.

THE TRICKY BUSINESS OF PACING

There are two important ways to think about pacing in your stories. The first is how to control time in storytelling. The second is to think about pacing as it manifests in sequencing, or in the breakdown of story into beats. Both are important, but we are going to give more of our attention to the latter, as it has a significant bearing on how you structure your screenplay overall.

Before we get started with that, however, let's spend a few moments thinking about pacing in terms of controlling time within scenes. Of course, directors, cinematographers, and editors use their crafts to influence the pace of storytelling. The coverage and the content of shots influence the rhythm of editing, but all these choices emerge from a close reading of your written story.

Scenes can be paced by the simple choice of when we enter and leave them. If the scene lands, or turns at a particular point, say at a line of dialogue, then ask yourself how much lead-in and pay-off you need for the story moment or moments to resonate. A fast-paced script takes chunks out of the opening and closing beats of a scene, so it gets to the point and moves on. A slower, more reflective story might allow scenes to build at a more leisurely pace.

We worked through an example of fast-paced description writing in *The Bourne Identity* in rule 8. This is just one example of how screenwriters write to accelerate pacing within a scene. The opposite tactic can be to fill a scene with the description of small but significant acts, like in this example from the shooting script of the character-led romantic drama *Leaving Las Vegas* (1995), written and directed by Mike Figgis.

```
INT. BEN'S BAR. LA - MORNING
```

```
The bar is dark but through a small window
we see that it is a very bright sunny day
outside. The bartender reads the Los Ange-
les Times. The bar surface is red vinyl.
There are five customers, all single men.
One of them is Ben and he is sitting at
the bar watching TV. A game show is in
progress and the TV sound is loud. Ben
finishes his drink and grimaces before
indicating to the barman that he'd like
a repeat. Barman pours him a whiskey-
cranberry -- and the camera moves in
closer to Ben, ending in a close-up. Ben
takes a big hit from the drink and con-
centrates on the TV. We hear from the TV
sound that it is a word game with a big
prize. Ben smiles to himself.
```

This scene uses a good many words although very little happens. And that's the point. We stick with it and fall into the rhythm of Ben's drinking. As a suicidal alcoholic, he does that a lot. The pacing alone is something of a character reveal. Remember that this kind of writing works when you have well-developed characters whose stasis resonates. It doesn't work when you are just filling pages with random stuff.

PACING YOUR STORY BEATS

Now let's turn to the pacing of beats within your story. In this book, we are working with a simple model of a feature-film story structure. That model is broken down into story beats, but not all beats are the same length or have the same importance in every story. Different stories will value different beats more highly and invest more pages—more time and, later, more money—into developing them. So, where one movie might skip through the debate beat in act one, another might play the beat longer.

For example, the debate beat in *Winter's Bone* is vital in establishing the opposition Ree Dolly will face in finding out what happened to her dad. She walks from isolated house to isolated house, being denied information at every turn. The beat is the longest in the movie, and, as we approach its end, we despair at Ree ever getting what she needs.

The longest beat in *How to Train Your Dragon* is the early progress beat in act two. It lasts more than twenty minutes and cuts back and forth between Hiccup bonding with and learning about his new friend, the dragon Toothless, and Hiccup applying what he has learned in warrior training in his village. This relationship between boy and dragon is the heart of the movie and we are given the time to enjoy watching it develop.

Both of these pacing choices work for their respective stories. But your story might put its emphasis somewhere else entirely. Every movie asks and answers the question of pacing on its own terms.

LINEAR PROGRESSION

Let's pick up on our scheme of story beats from rule 2, broken down into a little more detail. In a typical, linear, goal-driven story, it would look like this:

ACT ONE

PRIMARY EXPOSITION

STORY WORLD

This beat introduces our protagonist and embeds them in their world.

DESIRE

This beat clarifies our protagonist's starting goals and needs.

INCITING INCIDENT

It happens around here, either before or after the desire beat.

DEBATE

HESITATION

Our protagonist sees the difficulty in achieving their goals or has it pointed out to them.

FIRST COMMITMENT

They decide to try, nevertheless. But they are unprepared.

ACT TWO

EARLY PROGRESS

B STORY

A supporting character steps up to help. At this point help might not look like help!

PROGRESS

How far can your protagonist go without taking major risks or learning new skills?

RAISING STAKES

CHALLENGE

This is where things get significantly harder, pushing your protagonist toward . . .

DECISION

Now your protagonist is confronted by a real choice. Stop now or there's no going back.

MIDPOINT

Your protagonist chooses to commit fully to achieving their goals.

COMMITMENT

ACCELERATION

That commitment pays off right away with serious consequences. Things get harder . . .

... and harder still. But maybe the friends we made along the way can help.

CRISIS

CRISIS

Things are at their worst. Your protagonist is faced with extreme challenges. They are now the farthest away from achieving their goals they have ever been.

REVELATION

Or so it seems. Going through the crisis gives our protagonist (with the help of the B story character) clarity and purpose. Now they understand what they have to do, or are equipped to do it.

ACT THREE

CONFRONTATION

PLAN

Put the plan for victory into play.

PUSHBACK

The antagonist resists the plan, and we approach the final confrontation.

RESOLUTION

RESOLUTION

One side wins, and either way the movie's theme is resolved. Likely that means the protagonist achieves their goals in some way.

RESONANCE

The world of your story has changed. We may be given time to appreciate it.

Think of this sequence structure as a straw man. There are other ways of conceiving it, and I won't call the screenwriting police if you don't follow this structure. But it might be a useful reference if you are trying to keep on track writing a relatively mainstream movie. You'd be surprised how diverse a range of films follow exactly this kind of plan.

SAGE SPOTLIGHT:
WILLIAM GOLDMAN'S
TEN COMMANDMENTS

In his popular and entertaining book *Adventures in the Screen Trade: A Personal View of Hollywood and Screenwriting*, Goldman, screenwriter of *The Princess Bride* and *All the President's Men* (1976), offered his Ten Commandments for writers.

1. Thou shalt not take the crisis out of the protagonist's hands.
2. Thou shalt not make life easy for the protagonist.
3. Thou shalt not give exposition for exposition's sake.
4. Thou shalt not use false mystery or cheap surprise.
5. Thou shalt respect thy audience.
6. Thou shalt know thy world as God knows this one.
7. Thou shalt not complicate when complexity is better.
8. Thou shalt seek the end of the line, taking characters to the farthest depth of the conflict imaginable within the story's own realm of probability.
9. Thou shalt not write on the nose—put a subtext under every text.
10. Thou shalt rewrite.

WHY FRAGMENTED PROGRESSION IS STILL SEQUENTIAL

This is a big topic, but we'll start by discussing the use, and over-use, of a common cinematic storytelling device: the flashback. A flashback uses a past action to reveal something of significance to our story in the movie's present. Typically we flash back in a story in order to learn about a character's motivation and backstory, or to disentangle truth from perception. Used well and sparingly, flashbacks can be efficient alternatives to weighing down your scenes with expository dialogue, but flashbacks are also tricky because, when overdone, they can feel distracting or redundant rather than engrossing.

Expository Flashbacks

Writers need to trust their audience to extrapolate whole truths from partial information, and thus they shouldn't be too quick to rely on flashbacks. David Trottier, a screenwriter and author of *The Screenwriter's Bible*, has another warning about flashbacks: "We should not tell the reader about the past until that reader cares about the present." In most cases, I think that's excellent advice, although see the note on framing devices (page 143).

If you want to see how to write and direct flashbacks in an elegantly cinematic and narratively organic manner, Akira Kurosawa's innovative drama *Rashomon* (1950) uses multiple unreliable narrators giving evidence in court that we experience as flashbacks. *The Usual Suspects* (1995) revolves around the unreliable story told, in flashbacks, by Verbal Kint.

Although these movies tell their stories with complex and sometimes contradictory time shifts, they still conform to the tropes of classical movie storytelling. This includes the coherence of the sequence. For a more challenging deconstruction of time shifts, watch the remarkable horror-thriller *Don't Look Now* (1973). The movie uses memory, the irrational impetus of grief, and a subplot about the possibility of precognition to work its mysteries on the audience.

Framing Devices

Framing a movie by opening with a past event is not strictly a flashback, because there is no "present"—our contemporary characters have not yet emerged. It is worth mentioning here anyway, because using an opening event in a time before the present of your story can be a good way of avoiding the distracting nature of a true flashback and still getting expositional value from the past. You should still be judicious in using devices of this kind, because we are over-familiar with them.

When this kind of frame works well, as it does in Chris Marker's brilliant experimental science fiction narrative *La Jetée* (1962), it initiates a deeply resonant circularity to the movie. A violent incident remembered as a child is shown as a memory at the opening of the film. At the end of the film the incident is revealed to be the moment of the witness's death, in adulthood, in this dystopian story of time travel. The power of the storytelling is linked in part to its unity as a sequence. The encapsulated event plays out again as we realize what is about to happen again/for the first time. David Webb Peoples' screenplay for the Hollywood adaptation, *12 Monkeys* (1995), also uses this structure.

BREAKOUT STAR:
Quentin Tarantino on Structure and Narration (in 1994)

He's a big deal now, but here's Quentin Tarantino reflecting on story structure in his first produced screenplays during an interview with Gavin Smith for *Film Comment* in 1994:

"If you break it into three acts, the structure they all worked under was: in the first act the audience really doesn't understand what's going on, they're just getting to know the characters. The characters have far more information than the audience has. By the second act you start catching up and get even with the characters and then in the third act you now know far more than the characters know, you're way ahead of the characters. That was the structure *True Romance* was based on and you can totally apply that to *Reservoir Dogs*. In the first section, up until Mr. Orange shoots Mr. Blonde, the characters have far more information about what's going on than you have—and they have conflicting information. Then the Mr. Orange sequence happens and that's a great leveler . . . In the third part when you go back into the warehouse for the climax you are totally ahead of everybody."

In the Writers' Room:
SEQUENCING/MAPPING EXERCISE

Here you will outline the sequences that encapsulate your primary exposition beat. The exercise is in two parts: A and B. If you already have an outline for your current screenplay project, go straight to step B.

Step A: Map out the opening sequences of a movie in a prose outline in a straightforward linear fashion. Your outline will establish context for our protagonist—revealing the world they inhabit—and it will introduce their goals and needs. You will take us through the key events and images of the **story world** and **desire** beats (see page 36) so that by the end of your outline, your audience understands everything they need to follow your story. You should include an inciting incident within or at the end of these story beats, as appropriate for your story.

Here's a checklist of the things you will likely need to address:

1. Where and when is the movie set?
2. Who is your protagonist and what do they do?
3. What are their primary social and employment relationships?
4. How do they feel about their life, and how do you show this?
5. What is the one key thing they lack?
6. How does the inciting incident move their needs or goals forward, or impose challenges that explore their needs by other means?

CONTINUED ▶

Step B: Having done this, consider how a non-linear approach might change the way your story unfolds. You will still have to address the same questions, so much of the work you have already done will apply. Try some or all of these alternative methods to start your story. Work them all together in one version or in several iterations of the opening beats:

1. Start your movie with a past event as a prologue, or frame, setting up a context for what is about to happen in the present.
2. Include one or more flashbacks as an experiment, even if you are unsure this will fit your story.
3. Try integrating past, present, and even future events in a collage form, ordered by memory and thought rather than strict narrative logic. How does that new order affect the way your story is being told?

BE PURPOSEFUL IN YOUR DIALOGUE

Great lines punctuate great movies; they bring fans together across generations in their appreciation.

Some famous lines of dialogue have even come to represent entire movies in the popular imagination. For example, "I'll be back" from *The Terminator*, or "Rosebud" from *Citizen Kane* (1941).

Here's the irony around quotable movies and characters: Most of the important dialogue written for the screen goes unquoted because it is simple and doesn't draw attention to itself. It supports the drama, rather than leading it. That means it's doing its job.

Good dialogue emerges from character, from need, and from situation. If your dialogue supports and advances your drama without your audience being brought out of the story to pay attention to it, then you have done your job as a screenwriter.

Good dialogue is not about people talking as they do in real life. Strong dialogue is about people talking with purpose—with meaningful implication for their objectives and tactics.

START WITH RESEARCH

Every character is unique, and yet most fall into patterns of speech that reveal something about their background, their class, their education, their professional or work life, their gender, and their ethnicity. The way we speak and the words we use—or don't use—tell other people about us no matter what we are actually saying. If you are writing a character from Mobile, Alabama, they will have grown up with a particular way of speaking English that is different from somebody who grew up in London, England, or who learned English in high school in Latvia.

People adopt patterns of speech and expressions learned from their families, their friend groups, and their workplaces. Cops may have a way of speaking that uses work slang and shorthand, but New York cops and Los Angeles cops don't talk exactly alike. Some of these patterns of speech are shared and others represent an individual variation on a more general theme. Not every Londoner or Latvian speaks the same way—neither does a Londoner from Shakespeare's time or one from the year 2525.

When you need to be specific, do research. When you can't research, as with the example of a story set in the year 2525, then integrate speech patterns and vocabulary as a logical component of your story world creation.

Build Individuality

When you are comfortable that you know enough about how a character of a certain type and background would speak, then your next job is to make them sound like an individual. Your protagonist may be a fire-fighter, but he grew up in his unique family. He worked as a coal miner before changing jobs—that gives him a different kind of uniqueness. He is an amateur poet . . . he's an immigrant from Kenya . . . he's outgoing, and a bit of a joker. All these layers point you toward specificity.

Group Doesn't Equal Identical

Let's develop the quest for individuality further. I bet you and your group of school friends shared some colloquialisms without all sounding the same. Groups unify speech—they should feel like they are from the same place and time. However, they also give opportunities for you to signal individuality.

Who has the strongest accent in the group? Why? Who peppers their speech with the most pop culture references? Why? If you know your characters—if you have given them backstory, goals, wants, and needs—then you are already a long way toward answering those types of questions.

Here's an example of group banter from *Aliens* (1986). The colonial marines are waking up from hypersleep and grumbling like soldiers do. The dialogue in this science fiction movie draws our attention back in time to how we are trained to expect soldiers (in movies) to speak. Individuality will emerge from the pack, but in this scene it's all about establishing group speak.

```
GROANS echo across the chamber.

                    SPUNKMEYER
        Arrgh. I'm getting too old for this shit.

SPUNKMEYER says this sincerely, though he
must have enlisted underage not long ago.
Looking surly, DRAKE sits up. He's young
as well but street-tough. Nasty scar curl-
ing his lip into a sneer.

                    DRAKE
        They ain't payin' us enough for this.

                    DIETRICH
        Not enough to have to wake up to your
        face, Drake.

                    DRAKE
        Suck air. Hey, Hicks... you look
        like I feel.
```

SAGE SPOTLIGHT:
Shane Black on Writing Dialogue

We have already established that writing dialogue is not the same as writing people talking. In real life, our conversations are often rambling, full of non sequiturs, mumbling, and hesitation. In real conversations, the word "um" fights for dominance. Shane Black, writer of *Lethal Weapon* (1987) and *Iron Man 3* (2013), explains the difference between real conversations and Hollywood movie conversations:

"You can't write the way people actually talk in real life. You have to write the way they talk in movies and make it sound like it's real life . . . It's slightly heightened. Everything I do, I try to stylize it so that it's a little more interesting. A little more lively. It's a little bit more intense of a conversation."

BREAKING THE MOLD

People have always spoken in movies. Of course, until the coming of sound, we couldn't hear what they were saying. Sound brought with it new voices and new genres, notably the musical, and changed the rhythms and balance of storytelling in all motion pictures. It also gave opportunities to literary writers to bring their dialogue skills to moviemaking.

In some ways, classical Hollywood dialogue emerged out of that polyglot literary influence from journalists, novelists, and playwrights, and then became its own thing—concise, snappy, polished, and most of all, genre-driven. People spoke differently in a thriller than they did in a western or a comedy. Regional and class variations could also now be heard, and the talkies established those dialogue conventions that persist to this day.

In the 1960s and 1970s, the influence of method acting and new forms of European cinema (notably the French New Wave) scraped away at the classical polish. American movie dialogue moved further toward colloquialism, informality, and right up to the borders of incoherence (thank you, Marlon Brando). At the same time, new methods of recording dialogue influenced the way it would play in the sound mix. Robert Altman pioneered the use of radio mics, for example, and the "realistic" use of overlapping dialogue became more common.

Later innovations in dialogue writing sprang from independent movies. This forum gave screenwriters permission to innovate in the style of speechmaking. For example, you can find idiosyncratic and innovative speech patterns in most of the Coen brothers' movies, combining formality and informality, the use of highfalutin vocabulary in the middle of colloquial dialogue, and other techniques.

BREAKOUT STAR:
Andrew Haigh on Blocking

Although this is the element where we discuss dialogue, I thought this corrective from Andrew Haigh, writer/director of *Weekend* (2011) and *45 Years* (2015), was worth including. It's from an interview with Alex Heeney for Seventh Row. Haigh's comments speak to the importance of physical performance and staging—or blocking—as communication:

"Blocking is everything for me. In my head, when I'm working on a scene, the blocking always comes first. Especially when you're not cutting, you have to find that relationship between your camera and your characters. You have to develop that shot. You have to make it feel like there's some kind of progression. So blocking is absolutely essential. You can't make it all up on the day. You have to think a lot about it beforehand. I spend a lot of time trying to understand how Charley is going to walk into this room, and go to the fridge, and get to the table, and speak to the girlfriend who's in the house, and where is the dad going to come out, and how are they going to sit down. The minute you have any kind of longer take, you have to think about these things. I love how people exist within space and how they manage the space around them: how they feel comfortable in that space or embrace that space. So blocking can say a huge amount about character."

AVOIDING COMMON PITFALLS

Dialogue that is too literal, or that is saying exactly what your character means with no subtext, is what screenwriters call "on the nose." On-the-nose dialogue can feel redundant, telling us what we already know. Moreover, it can feel simplistic and unsatisfying. After all, human beings frequently avoid saying what they really think or feel, for all kinds of reasons. The true expression of feelings can be terrifying, inconvenient, embarrassing, inappropriate, or otherwise unwanted in any number of social and professional situations.

And yet sometimes being on the nose is the most appropriate, and most meaningful way you could possibly speak. Think of those three words: "I love you." Depending on the circumstances, that is either the tritest or the most eloquent thing you could possibly say. But maybe we want what we see in Cameron Crowe's *Say Anything* (1989) instead: John Cusack outside our window with a boombox held above his head playing "In Your Eyes." The lyrics of the song stand in for dialogue and the song is resonant because it was played on the night the two lovers first slept together, so, depending on your view of Peter Gabriel, that gesture could be more or less eloquent than *anything* the character could, in fact, *say*.

WHAT WE CAN LEARN FROM SILENT FILMS

When two characters meet, do they need to speak? Often the answer is "yes," but not always. Imagine the eloquent silence of two lovers strolling through the countryside together—two people so at home with one another that there is no need to fill the silence with small talk. Imagine a more terrible encounter, such as the long, slow revenge scene in Ingmar Bergman's *The Virgin Spring/Jungfrukällan* (1960). When Töre finds the goat herders who raped and murdered his daughter, he kills them without a word. Max von Sydow's performance communicates everything he is feeling with no need for dialogue until he is done, and the rage leaves him.

This brings us to a crucial point: Sometimes the best dialogue is none at all. Sometimes the most eloquent character in a scene is the one who is not talking. Think of Tom Hagen, the consigliere in *The Godfather* (1972). He is frequently present, and likely the smartest character in the room—especially when Sonny brings down the average—and yet, until called upon, he often keeps his own counsel. That doesn't mean we don't have a good idea what he's thinking. Robert Duvall is a fine actor, and his subtle reactions, including simple shifts of focus, are telling.

Cinema is a visual medium and you should never be afraid of letting images speak instead of words. Given that obvious piece of advice, ask yourself these questions:

- How are characters who are not speaking reacting to what is being said?
- How can I write around dialogue?
- How can I replace a line with a look or a shrug?

In the Writers' Room:
DIALOGUE EXERCISE

Here are three simple exercises to develop and test your dialogue skills.

TRANSCRIPTION

Here's a quick preparatory exercise. Record a real conversation between two people (who consent to be recorded) and transcribe it. Notice all of the starts and stops, the circularity, the hesitations, the diversions, the moments of excitement. That's not how movie dialogue works, and yet some of that might work, as character tactics, and some of it might be distilled down into voice.

STALLING

This exercise inserts conflict into the middle of a situation. Write a short scene where a character needs time, so they (creatively) stall. Figure out why they are stalling and give them at least three different tactics to do so that don't involve directly saying that they need time. Give the other character a good need also—what are they trying to get at? Give them three different tactics to get at what they want. Now your characters have needs and tactics. If they pursue them, you will have good dramatic conflict.

THE POWER OF SILENCE

Write a two-page scene with two characters. Both need something from the other, but only one speaks. How can the character who doesn't speak achieve their scene goals?

JUST FINISH YOUR FIRST DRAFT

You can read as many books and screenplays as you want to delay the inevitable. But if you want to be a screenwriter, you'll have to get used to this one unbreakable rule: Finish your draft.

Your job—as you have defined for yourself in purchasing this book—is to unlock the tools you need to finish your screenplay draft. For ten chapters now, we have looked more closely at the methods writers use to get there. Now we put them together to flesh out your draft.

As with so many screenwriting elements, there is no right or wrong way to get yourself to the finish line in the abstract. A productive method for one writer may be the demise of another. This chapter is really about confronting your own resistance and tricking yourself into completion. We'll start with some high-level strategies to spit out that draft, then lead into a list of tips to rely on when the going gets tough.

RELY ON—AND REFINE— YOUR OUTLINE

Keeping on track is really a function of keeping your ear to the ground in your story and being all over your outline. When something changes from your outline, and it will, you need to be able to make an informed judgment about that change. Do I shut it down? Do I go with it? Trust me, that's a choice you will have to make at some point as you write.

It doesn't matter how well you pre-plan your story. It doesn't matter how solid your outline is. As you write, new possibilities will open up. You'll turn a scene in a way you weren't anticipating, and it will lead to a new subplot, or new character choices. Your protagonist's boyfriend, who was underdeveloped in the outline because, well, you know, he's just the boyfriend, suddenly comes to life as you start to write his dialogue. Maybe he needs a bigger role. And so on and so on. This is good, this is healthy, just don't let it take you too far off course—unless it really starts to unravel your story in an inspirational way, and then it's back to the outline for you!

The truth is, if you do have an outline, you know where all your major scenes go, and hopefully all your minor ones as well. You know what happens in your story beats and sequences, and you know how they underpin your protagonist's arc or their progress toward their goals. If you know all this—or at least have a working version of all of it—then you really should be able to plow through to the end. If you don't, it's time to refine your outline.

LISTEN TO YOUR CHARACTERS

Working with characters is a little like walking an energetic dog. Allow yourself to be led by them, but always keep them on the leash. (In case you are losing the will to follow, the leash is your outline.) Your character-dogs will pull you in interesting directions and sniff out new ground—yes, we are committing to this analogy—but don't let them off the leash or they might get your story stuck down a sewer grate or under a truck.

If this is your first time writing a screenplay, the next statement might seem strange. If you are an old hand at creative writing, however, you will know exactly what I'm talking about: Your characters will start talking to you.

It's a fact. They will pipe up in your mind and tell you that they would or wouldn't do something that your story is asking them to. The better you know them, the more you will hear them speak in their own voice when you write their dialogue. They don't do it all the time, but you'll know them when you hear them. Sometimes you will know very clearly when you are trying to get them to say something that is out of character because you won't hear the lines in their voices.

REVISE AS YOU GO (WISELY!)

I read my way into the day's writing. And when I read, I revise, but only with discipline and in moderation. Revising small things—a line here, a description there—is fine if it gets you into being productive. I think of it as "tricking my way" into the day's writing. When I get to the blank page, I'm already writing so I just . . . continue. If you do this, take care not to fall into an endless loop of re-writing rather than making progress.

In general, making significant structural revisions as you're writing the script is unwise. If you come to a point where things really aren't working, then consider revising your outline first.

WRITE ACT ONE, THEN THE ENDING

This strategy tests your story by moving from premise to conclusion and then filling in the middle. If you can draft a first act, then you have set up everything important in your story.

Writing a first act means you have established your story world. You have placed your protagonist(s) within it in dramatic and emotional terms. You have established their wants, needs, and goals. You have introduced the antagonistic force and embodied it, in plot terms, usually in a character. You have established the beginning of a support network for your protagonists. You have written an inciting incident that sets the story on its path. You have highlighted the enormity of the challenge by dramatizing the protagonist's reluctance or concern in moving forward. You have set the initial terms for them to do so.

That's a lot of dramatic work. Those are also some big and very helpful signposts. If you move straight to the third act, the ending might already be in focus because if it. You can test out your premise by working on the ending. So why not just write it now? (If this is too hard—if you need to know exactly how act two feels before you can write act three—feel free to ignore this advice.

TRY A FLASH DRAFT

A flash draft is a sprint from wherever you are *now* to the end of the script. Don't stop. Don't read back. Don't revise. Not even for grammar and syntax. Not even to change that one thing you know you did wrong and is really ticking you off. Use that anger as an incentive to finish because *then*—and only then—you can correct it. Once again, for those of you with relatively little experience in screenwriting, this is the method I'd try first. If it doesn't work, by all means change the plan.

Having said that, a flash draft will be so much easier if you have done your prep first. I know I'm repeating myself again, but outline, outline, outline. If you don't believe me, read how Joss Whedon, the creator of *Firefly*, talks about his prep:

"Structure means knowing where you're going; making sure you don't meander about. Some great films have been made by meandering people, like Terrence Malick and Robert Altman, but it's not as well done today and I don't recommend it. I'm a structure nut. I actually make charts. Where are the jokes? The thrills? The romance? Who knows what, and when? You need these things to happen at the right times, and that's what you build your structure around: the way you want your audience to feel. Charts, graphs, colored pens, anything that means you don't go in blind is useful."

WHEN YOU WANT TO QUIT, TRY THESE

Lean into habit. When you want to quit, lean into habit. Ideally, you'll write every day. But "writing," of course, can mean different things. That might mean writing pages. It might also mean researching something that you will include in what you write later. It might mean sitting in a coffee bar and taking notes or watching a movie that inspires you. It might mean thinking about how you can steal from said movie to address some problem you're having. When you're facing a block or stifled by your own crippling expectations, focus on the routine rather than the outcome.

Bite off digestible chunks. A page is progress. A longer scene is more progress. This is one of those "look after the cents and the dollars take care of themselves" pieces of advice. If you think of the full 120 pages that you need to write when you are still writing your title page, that's a little bit terrifying. If you focus on the achievable, however, then the fear recedes. It never entirely goes away, but then a little fear is healthy.

Set achievable intermediate goals. This is just a step up from the previous note. Scenes lead to sequences, sequences to beats, and beats to acts. Give yourself a deadline of X days to write Y amount of your script. Don't be disappointed if you don't make the first deadline, just adjust your sights. It takes a while to learn what you can expect of yourself from day to day. Don't be unreasonable to yourself: Remember that some parts of the story are likely to be harder to write, and that some sequences will be longer than others. Give yourself flexibility but keep pushing forward.

End the day having started the next scene. This is a rule I swear by. Let's say you finish a scene and feel like you've really achieved something at the end of your writing day. Well, first of all, you have. Good for you. That's one less scene you have to draft—and maybe you actually wrote two scenes, or more. That's great. Well, the best way to celebrate, before you settle down with a snack and your over-affectionate dog on the couch, is to start the next scene. Write your slugline. Start the description. Write a few possible lines of dialogue. How about sketching in a line that sells the first scene beat? Leave yourself some notes: "Shelby asks for the divorce," or "Jerome tells Lydia about the ham sandwich," or "remember that Jeffrey can't see Veronica feeding his hamster behind his back," or whatever. Then the next day you can pick up those notes and hit the ground running.

Don't be afraid to write scenes or short sections out of sequence. If you are worried about a big scene that's coming up and you want to see how it can work, try it. If you need to know how something happens in order to plan how to get up to it, try it. Here we're talking about writing ahead on a much smaller scale than the write-your-ending method we set out above.

If something big changes, work the change into your outline before moving on. This is the one important exception to the flash draft rule. Don't worry about tiny changes, but if you get inspired or think you have found a better solution to a significant character or plot problem, then work it into your outline to test it out and to revise your plan before you commit too far to it in your script.

Give yourself permission to be imperfect. However good a writer you are, your first draft won't be perfect. This is especially true of dialogue, even more so of the dialogue you write in act one before you have truly found the voice of most of your characters. That's fine. Every writer writes sketchy dialogue in places in their first draft. The key is to make each scene do its job in terms of structural storytelling, and that includes having dialogue work to that goal. You are going to polish everything later anyway. Here's what Joss Whedon says—did I mention he was the creator of *Firefly*? Anyway, here's what he says about perfection in a first draft: "I have so many friends who have written two-thirds of a screenplay, and then re-written it for about three years . . . Even if it's not perfect, even if you know you're gonna have to go back into it, type to the end. You have to have a little closure."

Don't give in to doubt. Because you will doubt yourself, frequently and deeply, as you write. This is annoying, dispiriting, and completely normal. Every writer doubts their own work, even the great ones. Apart from that one guy, but we hate that one guy, right? Also, he's lying.

Don't worry if your first draft writes long. This is completely normal as well. It is much more common for first drafts to run long rather than short. If you are aiming for 100 to 110 pages and your first draft is 130, it's not the end of the world. Revision is 50 percent changing and 50 percent cutting, so it will come down by a significant amount.

In the Writers' Room:
DRAFTING EXERCISE

This exercise revolves around creating and sticking to a drafting routine. Follow these four steps to complete your first draft. (Remember, from here we'll head into revisions.)

First: Make a list of all the tasks that are part of the writing process. That includes writing scenes, but also researching, taking notes, writing character backstories, and so forth. When you have your list, print it out and make sure you do one or more of those things every day.

Second: Make a writing schedule. If you can find the same period of time every day, then set that aside. If your life is too complex for that—if it's anything like mine—then get out your calendar and book times for yourself that you can't or won't double-book.

Third: Set intermediate deadlines. Make a schedule of scenes, sequences, beats, and acts, assigning deadlines to some or all of them. You may change it, but now you have goals to work toward.

Fourth: Plan the treat you get for finishing your draft. I'm serious. Decide what you get when you're done. An expensive bottle of booze. A really nice meal out. A trip to see friends. All the ice cream. You're the creative—just be sure to make it something you really enjoy and deny yourself that reward until you are done with your draft.

Now hop over your resistance and write.

REVISE, REVISE, REVISE

Congratulations! You got to the end of your story. Now the work begins.

The first thing to say is this, and it might sound disappointing when you just got to the end: You don't really have a first draft yet. You still have a number of fairly straightforward tasks to perform before you can call yourself done with your initial draft and be ready for real revisions. We'll list a bunch of them quickly to get us up to speed. Do you know where the find/replace function is in your screenwriting software? Well, now's the time to find it.

Your initial rewriting tasks come in two sections. The first group is fairly technical, and the second requires a little more creative thought.

TECHNICAL CHECKS

If your second draft is remodeling, these tasks are like housework. They aren't going to put a new island in your kitchen, but they are going to do the washing up and clearing so that your kitchen is ready for its new look. Does that analogy work? Maybe . . . The point is that these tasks are important because they result in your first draft looking—and more importantly reading—like a unified whole and not the weird Frankenstein creation born of waves of contradictory inspiration and the occasional bad idea.

Spelling and Grammar Check

This one is obvious. Go back through the screenplay and correct all the errors and awkward constructions you left behind in the wake of your frenzied typing. Don't be embarrassed, everyone does it. I literally just typed embarrassed as "embarrassesdd," and now I've done it again and my spell check is disappointed in me. Look, the occasional typo is fine; nobody's perfect. Just don't be a slacker, because if you give me your screenplay to read and there are multiple spelling mistakes in the first two pages, then I'm going to conclude either that you can't write or that you are a lazy writer who has no respect for me as a reader. Neither conclusion is your friend.

Format Check

The same applies to screenplay format. You don't have to be perfect, and you don't have to be bland. You can display your style in part though creatively working around some of the rules of format. But if I can't follow the action in your scenes and you waste my time trying to figure out why your messy script looks the way it does, then you are going to lose my goodwill very fast. Take a pass to smarten up your formatting.

Consistency Check

Did a character's name change? Did their gender change? Or their age? Did you rename a location halfway through act two, or change the antagonist's military rank? There are so many things that shift around or go back and forth when you write a screenplay. Some are small things, some very big, but all of them need to be consistent. Take a pass through, just making sure that you have actioned them all. I told you find/replace was going to be important, right?

"Show, Don't Tell" Check

You remember that basic screenwriting maxim? Well, inevitably some "show, don't tell" fails will have crept into your screenplay without you realizing it. This happens to everyone. So take a pass just asking yourself if you are breaking the rule that says we can't access a character's internal thoughts just through description.

CREATIVE CHECKS

Having spruced things up, now we are going to take a couple more passes through the draft looking for ways to get the most value and consistency out of your action descriptions and your dialogue. Again, these stages are not a full rewrite. You are not messing significantly with your story structure, with character development, or with the order of scenes and sequences. Rather you are going to search for *narrative economy*—how to say more with fewer words—and to make sure that your characters sound the same at the beginning as they do at the end.

Description Peel

For this pass, you need to examine every action description in your screenplay and ask yourself whether it is over-written. We have already discussed how to write action in a screenplay, and you can use those guidelines to help you through.

For each scene, ask yourself the following questions:

- Can I say the same thing, just as eloquently, with fewer words?
- If there are big paragraphs, can I break up the text into thought images and use more white space without taking significantly more space on the page?
- Am I repeating something in action that is also covered in dialogue, or vice versa?

The ideal end result is eloquent scenes that may not take up less page space but make for a faster and easier read by using shorter statements and more white space. Having said that, you can probably cut at least ten pages from your screenplay through this single step alone. The acronym to follow is ABC = Always Be Cutting.

Editing Dialogue

We talked about how you write your way into dialogue as you get to know a character better in rule 10. Well, this pass is all about correcting for any evolution in your own understanding of the characters.

Some questions to live by:

- How does a character sound at the start of the story?
- How do they sound at the end?
- If there is a significant difference between the two, ask yourself: Does the difference emerge organically from character change, or arbitrarily from the way I am writing the character? If the latter, then you have some work to do.

Once you have dealt with all those issues, you have a working first draft. Now it's time to revise.

TROUBLESHOOTING YOUR SCRIPT

Revision is a huge topic, and all we can hope to do here is to remind you of the kind of things writers often do when they approach revisions.

First, Do No Harm

Save a version of your script as it was before you start revising. You want a clean version of each draft so you can go back to it for purposes of comparison, or because you might like the original version of a scene or a speech better and want to revert at some point. Date your development drafts and number them to make it easy to find what you need in the future.

Next, Take It One Task at a Time

Make sure you have clear goals for a rewrite task. Just like the technical passes we outlined above, have a single purpose. Your more substantial rewrite tasks should be planned and targeted as much as possible in advance. Pick one lead issue and work it until it is fixed and then move on to the next.

If you think your script has problems in the relationship between the protagonist and their mentor, the climax needs punching up, and you feel things lag between pages 51 and 57, address them one at a time. Solve one and move on. Of course, sometimes—often—issues overlap, but the principle still holds.

Common Issues

Typical script problems emerge from plot, character, or concept, or from some combination thereof. You thought things made sense when you were writing your outline, but now . . . not so much. Here are a few straightforward options for all three.

Plot and Story Problems

There are many potential problems to consider, but here are three common ones. These are important because they have a huge bearing on the rest of the story.

Is it the inciting incident? Maybe your story needs a different or stronger way to start. Does your incident establish or direct goals, needs, and wants? If not, beef it up or change it.

Is it act two? Hint: It's usually act two. Your story starts okay, but then it bogs down. Are things too passive? Beef up your antagonist and push your characters harder. Does your midpoint change the game? If not, beef it up. Is your crisis really a crisis—will your protagonist never be the same again? If not . . . well you know the score by now, and you also know that I love to use "beef" as a verb.

Is it the climax? Does your climax effectively resolve your story's theme and your protagonist's arc? Is it exciting enough, or dramatically satisfying? Has the world of your story changed in a significant, if possibly subtle way because of the story you are telling? If not, then act three needs work.

SAGE SPOTLIGHT:
John August on Revising

On his blog, American screenwriter John August offers similar advice on how to approach revisions. He also recommends working with a printed version of your script. That's essential for me, as it happens. I always notice things on the printed page that I never do on the screen:

"The biggest problem with most rewrites is that you start at page one, which is already probably the best-written page in the script. You tweak as you go, page after page, moving commas and enjoying your cleverness—all the while forgetting why you're rewriting the script. Instead, you need to stop thinking of words and pages, and focus on goals. Are you trying to increase the rivalry between Helen and Chip? Then look through the script—actual printed script, not the one onscreen—and find the scenes with Helen and Chip. Figure out what could be changed in those scenes to meet your objectives. Then look for other scenes that help support the idea. Scribble on the paper. Scratch out lines. Write new ones. Then move on to your next goal. And your next one."

Character Problems

If your characters won't behave, or they seem inconsistent, then you are probably making them do things they don't want to do. You created them; you set up the rules and parameters for their behavior. That means you can change those rules and parameters. When there is friction, either you are right, and you need to change the characters to fit the story, or they are right, and you need to need to change the story so it fits the characters. Either way, you need to go back to your outline and to act one and take another look at their arcs.

Conceptual Issues

Stories can't do everything, and they can't be about everything—not in 120 pages. A common problem is that writers expect their stories to carry a whole lot of symbolic water that they simply are not capable of carrying. Remember ABC? Often scripts need a bit of conceptual trimming after a first draft. You tried to squeeze everything in but now you need to cut a whole lot of material out. Ask yourself: What is core and what is peripheral? As screenwriters say: Kill your darlings.

WHAT ROLE DO COLLABORATORS, MENTORS, AND READERS PLAY?

Writers often like to think of themselves as solo acts, but in reality, screenwriters write for a large audience. With that in mind, you might seek out your own test audience to help you in your writing and revising process. Here are some of the people who might work with you to make your screenplay better:

Collaborators

Many great writers work in teams. If you can find somebody who gets you, and whose skills complement your own, then they might be a potential collaborator. Be careful here, because there are many pitfalls in co-writing. Just because somebody is a good friend doesn't mean they are the right person for you to go into a writing partnership with. Indeed, many friendships are tested or even ruined that way.

If you are thinking about writing with another person, I would suggest that you start by testing out the relationship with a small project, or a small step in the development of a larger one. Give yourselves the opportunity to back out before things get too involved. If you do find someone to collaborate with, remember to put together and sign a *Writers' Collaboration Agreement*. This is a simple legal document that sets up who owns what in the creative partnership and who does what in the team. You can find boilerplate models online that are pretty much ready to go. Keep a copy for your records.

Mentors

Do you know anyone whose opinion on your screenplay is likely to be well informed? Do you have family, friends, or college professors who are connected to the movie business? If you do, then now might be the time politely to approach them, as long as you have a real relationship or connection and not merely a brief professional association.

Warning: If you are working as a production assistant (or similar) and you have just met a producer, now is NOT the time to ask them to read your script. Unless they ask for it. Which they won't. At least not until they know you better and respect you.

Similarly, be careful about joining a writers' group. Not all groups are the same. Some are deeply toxic, or merely uninformed or unhelpful. However, if you can find one that fits and you can get valuable feedback from a range of different voices and perspectives, then a group can be immensely valuable. One piece of advice here: Be cold-blooded about it; if and when the group doesn't work for you, leave immediately. Participating in this group should be primarily a professional—not a social—activity. The people in the group deserve your respect and their work deserves your attention, until you or they have nothing useful to contribute.

Readers

This is by no means a requirement, but you might consider employing a professional script reader to give feedback on your screenplay. Typically, this kind of feedback comes in the form of detailed notes, or a coverage report outlining strengths, weaknesses, and suggestions for improvement. The advantage of using a professional is that you are going to get the kind of notes and responses that your script would get from an average agency, producer, or studio. In other words: fairly predictable mainstream responses. If you are not writing a mainstream movie, then think carefully about how useful such a reading will be for you.

When to Hire a Script Reader

Option One: After your first draft If you have finished a draft—including all the checks, dialogue edits, the description peel, and you have been through your structure and neatened up the arcs and beats—then you could be ready for someone to read your script. Having a professional reading at this point is probably more valuable if you have just finished your first screenplay, because it likely will highlight all the things you need to do in your second draft.

Option Two: After your second draft If this isn't your first attempt at writing a screenplay, then I would normally recommend that you undertake at least two proper drafts before you bring in a professional reader. Your second draft anticipates the notes your first draft would have merited and corrects the things your experience already tells you need correcting. Then a reader comes in with a fresh eye, and that can be helpful.

Option Three: Never—or . . . Unless you really trust the person to give you what you need, don't hire them. Bad notes can be destructive both in terms of clarifying what needs work and in terms of your morale as a writer. By "bad notes," I don't just mean critical responses—if you are a writer, you need to develop a thick skin. No, what I mean is notes that are unhelpful. There are a lot of poor readers out there and, unless you know them personally or trust recommendations, it's a bit of a gamble.

In my opinion, if you are just starting out, it's much better to pay a professional to read your screenplay and meet with you to discuss it than to write a general coverage report or send you notes. If they charge a little more for a meet-up, I say it's worth paying. When I consult on screenplays, as I do regularly, I prefer to meet in person with an inexperienced writer for a couple of hours. I find that my notes don't always land in the way I intend with somebody who hasn't been through the process and, given that all writers see things differently, it helps to be able to discuss things in person. "In person" can mean online via a Zoom meeting or similar service, of course.

Finding a good reader can be tricky. Word of mouth is always useful. If friends or colleagues have used somebody and rave about them, that's a good start. Similarly, if you can find somebody who specializes in the kind of story you are telling, that might be a good place to start. Picking a random name out from the Internet is a lottery.

In the Writers' Room:
REVISION EXERCISE

THE ARC MARKUP

In this exercise, we are going to check whether you have actually done what you planned to do. I want you to read through your screenplay *without reference to your outline* and make notes every time your protagonist's arc develops. Every time they act on their theme or undergo a moment of character development, make a note. At the end of your read, you should have a series of bullet points. Now read through them in relation to your outline or beat sheet. Do they conform? If not, why not? Now you have to decide which version is better and make revision plans accordingly.

WHAT'S NEXT?

You did it. You now have a solid draft and that's a significant achievement. You are well on the way to having a producible property. But you are probably going to need to revisit your script several more times if you want to sharpen it for submission, let alone to take it into production. What follows is aimed primarily at those of you who are starting out and who don't, as yet, have contacts in the movie business.

There are many things you can do to move your career forward but, as an aspiring screenwriter, you need to get your screenplays read. That's tricky, unless you have a track record, which is to say "a reason why someone might want to read your writing." What I'm going to do is to lay out a few notes about how things work and how you can move forward. This isn't the only path, but it will help focus your thinking if nothing else.

KNOW THE BUSINESS

Whatever else you do, now is the time to start researching the business. You can read the trades and the coverage of the industry in news outlets. Start with free online trades and see how you are doing. The trades are a guide to what's going on. You will start to care about general trends, innovations, industrial disputes, and developments in distribution among other topics. Everything adds to your awareness of what the industry is thinking about and responding to at the moment. Being up-to-date on the latest events doesn't mean anyone will buy your script, but it does mean you can hold an informed conversation with your fellow professionals, and that's a start.

You can also use search engines creatively and read up on screenwriting advice. There are spec sales trackers that log every screenplay that is sold; don't be fooled out of writing what you want to write, but trackers will give you a sense of what's selling now. That's not necessarily the same as what will be selling next month, so don't fret about it. You could start by checking out Script Pipeline (scriptpipeline.com/category/script-sales). There is an abundance of other options, but you could do worse than following some of the links from the Additional Resources section of this book. Remember to take a look at the Black List—it's a good place to start (blcklst.com). At least, it was when I wrote this book!

Agents and/or managers are also important for a professional screenwriter but, once again, they won't be interested in you until you give them a reason to be. That means you need a track record.

GETTING A TRACK RECORD

For movie screenwriters (TV is its own thing and we're not covering that here), there are a number of valid options for getting a track record. Some of them you can do from anywhere, while others require you to be where movies get made. Often, but not always, that means living in Southern California. Here are some pointers:

Work Freelance

If you want to open doors, meet the people behind those doors. One of the best ways to do that is to work for and with them. Get a job on set as a production assistant (if necessary, network to find someone who will take you on) or use any skills you may have learned at film school or elsewhere to get freelance gigs. Talk to your co-workers. Be the kind of person they want to have around. That will get you employed by the same people again. Eventually, you will meet people who will be interested in helping you move forward. There's a useful article in IndieWire by Barbara Freedman Doyle that will set you straight on how to make your freelancing pay off and how to avoid shooting yourself in the foot. It's called "The Six Things You Must Know to Make it in the Film Industry." You can find it here: indiewire.com/2012/04/the-six-things-you-must-know-to-make-it -in-the-film-industry.

Go Network

The movies are a relationship-driven business. The more people in the business you meet, the more likely it is that you will find someone who can be helpful to you. Be aware that many relationships in movies are to a certain extent contingent. Everyone is looking for something from someone else. Also be aware that professional relationships are as much about history as they are about actual friendship. What have you done together? Having said that, there are a great many lovely people who work in movies. You should try and meet as many of them as you can, socially and professionally. One good place to network with movie people is at film festivals, but don't expect to be chatting with the elite of the industry in their roped-off VIP areas.

Enter Competitions

There are lots of screenwriting competitions, many of which are exclusively aimed at unproduced screenwriters. Some competitions are open, others have genre categories or are only for certain kinds of screenplays or screenwriters: a theme, a gender, a genre. They are of differing levels of renown, but success in any competition is worth something. If your script wins or is a finalist in a number of competitions, that's the beginning of a track record.

Make the Movie

If you make short films or microbudget features that get screened and even win prizes at festivals, welcome to a track record. Making shorts with technical support is one reason people go to film school.

Go to Film School

It is worth considering film school if you have the resources and if you can find a program that feels right for you. There are numerous screenwriting programs at the undergraduate and MFA levels, but most general film programs—like the ones I teach for at the School of Cinema in San Francisco State University—include screenwriting as an important part of their curriculum. I don't want to bite the hand that feeds me, but I will add that you really don't *need* to go to film school to write a meaningful or profitable screenplay. The long and the short of it is that you need to find ways to make connections and prove your potential.

THE END

The world will never run out of stories to tell and fortunately the craft of screenwriting costs very little to practice. When you have written one screenplay, it will be easier to write the next. Frankly, the next one is also likely to be better because now you know what you are doing, right? The bottom line, if you want to be a professional screenwriter the only rule that really matters is this one:

Keep writing.

Additional Resources

ON AGENTS, MANAGERS, AND THE BUSINESS OF SCREENWRITING

Andy Rose, *The Aspiring Screenwriter's Dirty Lowdown Guide to Fame and Fortune*. New York: St. Martin's Press, 2018.

ON ARCHETYPES

Christopher Vogler, *The Writer's Journey: Mythic Structure for Writers, Third Edition*. Studio City, CA: Michael Wiese Productions, 2007.

John Truby, *The Anatomy of Story: 22 Steps to Becoming a Master Storyteller*. New York: Faber & Faber, 2007.

ON EXPERIMENTAL SCREENWRITING

Scott MacDonald, *Screen Writings: Scripts and Texts by Independent Filmmakers*. Berkeley, CA: University of California Press, 1995.

ON FORMATTING

Christopher Riley, *The Hollywood Standard: The Complete & Authoritative Guide to Script Format and Style, 2nd Edition*. Studio City, CA: Michael Wiese Productions, 2009.

David Trottier, *The Screenwriter's Bible, 7th Edition, A Complete Guide to Writing, Formatting, and Selling Your Script*. West Hollywood, CA: Silman-James Press, 2019.

ON THE HISTORY OF SCREENWRITING

Andrew Horton and Julian Hoxter, editors, *Screenwriting (Behind the Silver Screen Series, Book 8)*. New Brunswick, NJ: Rutgers University Press, 2014.

Marc Norman, *What Happens Next: A History of American Screenwriting*. New York: Three Rivers Press, 2007.

Steven Maras, *Screenwriting: History, Theory, Practice*. New York: Wallflower Press, 2009.

Steven Price, *A History of the Screenplay*. London: Palgrave Mac-Millan, 2013.

ON INDEPENDENT SCREENWRITING

J. J. Murphy, *Me and You and Memento and Fargo*. New York: Continuum, 2007.

Ken Dancyger and Jeff Rush, *Alternative Scriptwriting: Beyond the Hollywood Formula, 5th Edition*. Abingdon, Oxon: Focal Press, 2013.

ON SCREENWRITING IN THE CONTEMPORARY MEDIA INDUSTRIES

Daniel Bernardi and Julian Hoxter, *Off the Page: Screenwriting in the Era of Media Convergence.* Oakland, CA: University of California Press, 2017.

SCREENWRITING SOFTWARE (SELECTED)

CeltX: Celtx.com

Final Draft: Finaldraft.com

Movie Magic Screenwriter: Write-bros.com/movie-magic -screenwriter

Trelby (free): Trelby.org

ONLINE RESOURCES, PODCASTS, AND BLOGS

3rd & Fairfax (podcast of the Writers Guild of America West): WGA.org/3rdandfairfax

Go Into The Story (blog of the Black List): GoIntoTheStory .blcklst.com

Scriptnotes (John August's podcast): JohnAugust.com/podcast

Script Shadow (script reviews and more): ScriptShadow.net

The Writers Store: WritersStore.com

References

Anderson, L. V. "A Conversation with Lynn Shelton." Slate. June 18, 2012. slate.com/culture/2012/06/lynn-shelton-interview-the-your-sisters-sister-and-humpday-director-on-improvising-and-directing-mad-men.html

August, John. "Library." JohnAugust.com. Accessed February 20, 2019. johnaugust.com/library#bigfish

August, John. "How to Rewrite." JohnAugust.com. August 17, 2005. johnaugust.com/2005/how-to-rewrite

August, John. "How to Write a Scene, now in handy two-page form." JohnAugust.com. June 18, 2014. johnaugust.com/?s=how+to+write+a+scene

Brady, John. The Craft of the Screenwriter. New York: Simon and Schuster, 1982.

Bray, Catherine. "Joss Whedon's Top 10 Writing Tips." Aerogramme Writers' Studio, re-blogged from Hotdog magazine, original unavailable. March 13, 2013. aerogrammestudio.com/2013/03/13/joss-whedons-top-10-writing-tips

Bucher, John. "4 Horror Archetypes That Work in Any Genre." LA Screenwriter. May 13, 2015. la-screenwriter.com/2015/05/13/4-horror-archetypes-that-work-in-any-genre

Debruge, Peter. "Interview with Joe Swanberg." Variety. March 5, 2008. variety.com/2008/music/markets-festivals/interview-with-joe-swanberg-1117981936

Doyle, Barbara Freedman. "The Six Things You Must Know to Make it in the Film Industry," IndieWire. April 4, 2012. indiewire.com/2012/04/the-six-things-you-must-know-to-make-it-in-the-film-industry-48357

Ellis, Jennifer. "Female Character Archetypes and Strong Female Characters." JenniferEllis.ca. April 1, 2015. jenniferellis.ca/blog/2015/4/1/female-character-archetypes-and-strong-female-characters

Field, Syd. "Callie Khouri on creating character: Thelma and Louise." SydField.com. Accessed April 21, 2020. sydfield.com/syd_resources/callie-khouri-on-creating-character-thelma-louise

Field, Syd. Screenplay. New York: Bantam Dell, 1979.

Giroux, Jack. "'Get Out' Director Jordan Peele on his Filmmaking Debut & the Power of Story." Slash Film. posted February 24, 2017. slashfilm.com/get-out-jordan-peele-interview

Goldman, William. Adventures in the Screen Trade: A Personal View of Hollywood and Screenwriting. New York: Warner Books, 1983.

Heeney, Alex. "Andrew Haigh: 'Blocking is Everything.'" Seventh Row. April 16, 2018. seventh-row.com/2018/04/16/andrew-haigh-lean-on-pete

Hoxter, Julian. *Write What You Don't Know: An Accessible Manual for Screenwriters*. New York: Continuum Books, 2011.

Kaufman, Anthony. "Kicking and Screaming: Noah Baumbach Grows Up With 'Greenberg.'" IndieWire. March 18, 2010. indiewire.com/2010/03 /kicking-and-screaming-noah-baumbach-grows-up-with-greenberg-245576

Kroll, Noam. "How to Write the Perfect Logline: And Why It's As Important as Your Screenplay." IndieWire. January 6, 2014. indiewire.com/feature/how-to -write-the-perfect-logline-and-why-its-as-important-as-your-screenplay -31710

Lee, Michael. "Screenwriting Tips from Action Movie Screenwriter Shane Black: Part 1." The Script Lab. June 5, 2019. thescriptlab.com/features /screenwriting-101/10391-screenwriting-tips-from-action-movie -screenwriter-shane-black-part-1

Lewis, Kevin. "Robert Altman: The Sound Crew's Best Companion." *Cinemontage*. May 1, 2007. cinemontage.org/robert-altman

MacDonald, Scott. *Screen Writings: Scripts and Texts by Independent Filmmakers*. Berkeley, CA: University of California Press, 1995.

Mamet, David. *On Directing Film*. New York: Penguin, 1992.

Marchese, David. "Aaron Sorkin on how he would write the Democratic primary for 'The West Wing.'" *The New York Times*. March 2, 2020. nytimes.com /interactive/2020/03/02/magazine/aaron-sorkin-interview.html

Marks, Dara. *Inside Story: The Power of the Transformational Arc*. Studio City, CA: Three Mountain Press, 2007.

McKee, Robert. *Story: Substance, Structure, and the Principles of Screenwriting*. New York: Harper Collins, 1997.

Murphy, J. J. *Me and You and Memento and Fargo*. New York: Continuum, 2007.

Myers, Scott. "Screenwriting 101: Ava DuVernay." The Blacklist. July 25, 2017. gointothestory.blcklst.com/screenwriting-101-ava-duvernay-abcc5ee8e3be

Rodriguez, Ashley. "Keeping up with Netflix originals is basically a part-time job now." Quartz. January 1, 2019. qz.com/1505030/keeping-up-with -netflix-originals-is-basically-a-part-time-job-now

Rossio, Terry. "Treatment for *The Mask of Zorro*." Wordplay. Accessed April 21, 2020. wordplayer.com/columns/wp37-xtras/wp37x.ZORRO.html

Simon, Alex. "Forget It Bob, It's Chinatown: Robert Towne looks back on *Chinatown*'s 35th anniversary." The Hollywood Interview. February 1, 2009. thehollywoodinterview.blogspot.com/2009/10/robert-towne-hollywood -interview.html

Smith, Gavin. "Quentin Tarantino: 'When you know you're in good hands.'" *Film Comment*. July-August, 1994. filmcomment.com/article/quentin-tarantino-interviewed-by-gavin-smith

Snyder, Blake. *Save the Cat: The Last Book on Screenwriting You'll Ever Need*. Studio City, CA: Michael Wiese Productions, 2005.

Trottier, David. *The Screenwriter's Bible, 7th Edition, A Complete Guide to Writing, Formatting, and Selling Your Script*. West Hollywood, CA: Silman-James Press, 2019.

Truby, John. *The Anatomy of Story: 22 Steps to Becoming a Master Storyteller*. New York: Faber & Faber, 2007.

Vogler, Christopher. *The Writer's Journey: Mythic Structure for Writers, Third Edition*. Studio City, CA: Michael Wiese Productions, 2007.

Woolverton, Linda. "How we made Beauty and the Beast." *The Guardian*. March 13, 2017. theguardian.com/culture/2017/mar/13/how-we-made-beauty-and-the-beast

Writers Store. "Interview with John Truby." Accessed April 21, 2020. writersstore.com/interview-with-john-truby

Zacharias, Ramona. "Damien Chazelle on La La Land." Creative Screenwriting. February 10, 2017. creativescreenwriting.com/la-la-land

WRITERS GUILD OF AMERICA REPORTS

2019 WGAW Annual Report to Writers: wga.org/the-guild/about-us/annual-report

Writers Guild of America West Issues Inclusion Report Card for 2017-18 TV Staffing Season: wga.org/news-events/news/press/2019/wgaw-issues-inclusion-report-card-for-2017-18-tv-staffing-season

SCREENPLAYS DIRECTLY QUOTED

500 Days of Summer (2009) by Scott Neustadter & Michael H. Weber

Aliens (1986) by James Cameron

Bonnie and Clyde (1967) by David Newman & Robert Benton

The Bourne Identity (2002) by Tony Gilroy

La La Land (2016) by Damien Chazelle

Leaving Las Vegas (1994) by Mike Figgis

Lost in Translation (2003) by Sofia Coppola

The Princess Bride (1987) by William Goldman

Terminator Salvation (2005) by John Brancato & Michael Ferris

War of the Worlds (2005) by John Friedman and David Koepp

Index

About the Author

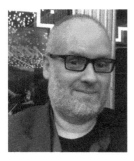

Julian Hoxter is an associate professor in the School of Cinema at San Francisco State University. He is also the screenwriting coordinator at SFSU and has taught and practiced screenwriting for over 20 years. Hoxter is a produced screenwriter and a professional script consultant. His screenplays have won three competitions and have been finalists in many more. Over the course of his career, he has written a number of textbooks on screenwriting, as well as scholarly volumes on screenwriting history and on the contemporary media industries.

CPSIA information can be obtained
at www.ICGtesting.com
Printed in the USA
JSHW031543280720
6969JS00002B/5